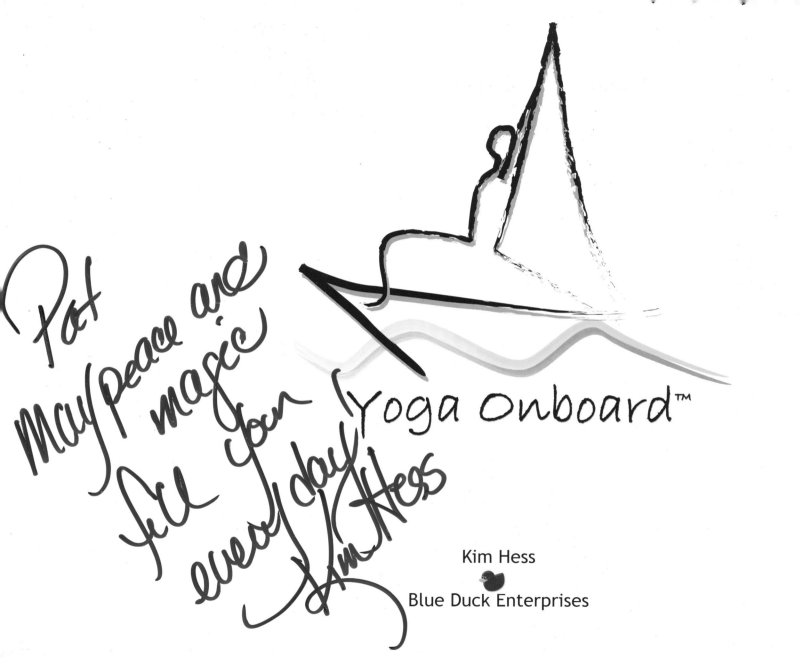

Pat

May peace and
magic
fill your
everyday

Yoga Onboard™

Kim Hess

Blue Duck Enterprises

MW01039828

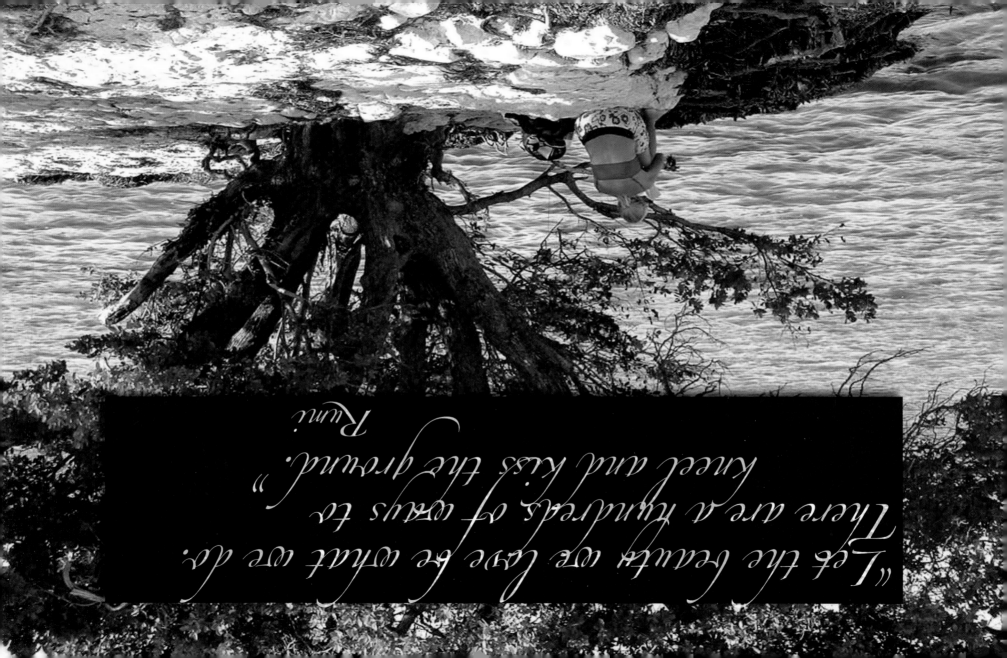

"Let the beauty we love be what we do.
There are hundreds of ways to
kneel and kiss the ground."

Rumi

Congratulations on choosing to incorporate a yoga practice into your live-aboard lifestyle!
By building an awareness of your body, your thought process and your breath,
you will be able to tap into a creative source that will enable you to
expand your practice beyond what you see here.

Namaste,

Kim

Yoga is..."the oldest system of personal development in the world,
encompassing body, mind and spirit."
BKS Iyengar

Table of Contents

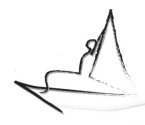

Table of Contents

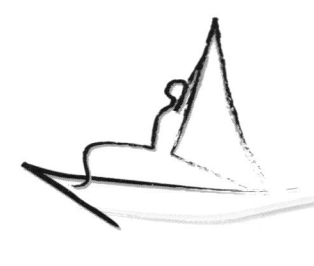

Foreword
by Melanie Neale

When you think about it, life aboard a boat is like practicing yoga every day. We walk around the deck ducking slightly to avoid hitting the shrouds. We place our feet a certain distance apart so that our balance is optimized. And we do these things without thinking about them.

But what if we were to think a little bit more about what we do every day? What if we took the teachings of yoga and applied them to the way we walk to the bow of the boat to lift the anchor, or the way we throw our bodies into raising the sails? What if, every time we did something, we strove to do it more conscientiously?

I met Kim Hess through a yoga instructor and friend who I'd been practicing with for a few years. My friend told me that I had to meet Kim, because we were both sailors and both dedicated to the cruising life. Kim was a yoga instructor who was developing a program and writing a book about adapting a yoga practice to the live-aboard lifestyle, and I was a live-aboard sailor and writer who loved yoga. I knew we needed to meet. So, I asked Kim to help me move.

Short Story, the 28' Columbia sailboat that I'd lived aboard for almost five years, sailing on the weekends and whenever I could, had to be moved from her home base in North Miami to a new marina in Dania, Florida. I was leaving a group of people that I'd come to love, and was taking only my boat, my boyfriend and my dog with me. I knew it was going to be hard, because leaving a home always is, but as soon as we cleared the dock and pointed Short Story's bow out to open water, Kim and I started playing with different poses on the deck and I knew everything was going to be okay.

From that day on, any chance to go sailing became a chance to practice yoga. On a short cruise in Lake Superior aboard Trillium, a Tartan 34, I discovered something that I had always suspected but never felt: a boat has its own energy, and if you take the energy that your body and soul produce while practicing yoga and combine it with a boat's energy, you'll feel more connected to the boat and the ocean and everything around you than you ever have before.

A boat takes energy in from nature. The wind foils around a sail, centering on a certain point or center of balance in the sail and pushing downward. The downward motion of the wind energy is what makes the boat move. Most people think that sailboats are simply pushed by the wind, but this isn't true. They are designed to harness the wind's energy, funnel it downward through the mast, and spread it through the boat's hull and into the water. This is a non-technical explanation of something that makes more sense in a book on yacht design, but it relates to yoga in more ways that we can imagine.

While on Lake Superior, sailing aboard Trillium, I experienced the perfect combination of a body's energy with a boat's. First, I did a few casual inversions with my feet against the boom. Then standing on the cabin top, I stood in warrior one. My feet lined up with the boom and I rested my hip against it. On impulse, I leaned my body into the sail. I was on the windward side of the boat, so I was able to lean far enough to give all the muscles along my side a significant stretch. As I leaned into the sail, my fingers touched it. Then my arm and my ribcage came to rest against it. The wind hummed through the sail and I felt the energy moving through me and downward to my feet, which were planted on Trillium's deck, then through them and into the fiberglass cabin. At the same time, my own prana was moving upwards through my body and into the sails, not moving against the wind's energy, but complementing it.

I truly believe that there is nothing else like this book. Many books have been written about boats and many have been written about yoga, but the two have never been combined. If this book gives you one thing, and I think it will give you many, it should be the freedom to let your imagination guide your yoga practice. A yoga practice is not rigid: it can change from boat to boat and from ocean to ocean. Let your boat, your capabilities and your mood shape your practice, and let Yoga Onboard be your teacher.

Melanie Neale, s/v Short Story
Dania Beach, Florida

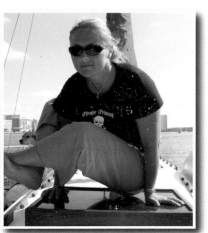

"Each friend represents a world in us, a world possibly not born until they arrive, and it is only by this meeting that a new world is born."
Anais Nin

A Seed was Planted

The first time I lived on a boat – a 42' Tayana - I had just completed my yoga teacher training. The first couple of weeks I enjoyed practicing on the dock near our slip. Once we left our slip to sail through the Keys for a month, I found myself adapting my practice to life on the boat. There was not a single flat place on the vessel that was big enough for me to lay down my mat. I practiced forward folds in the cockpit, meditated on the bow and created new and exciting standing postures while holding onto a cross bar on the stern, all this being done both under sail or on the hook, the heeling or the stillness creating the perfect practice for that particular day.

Once I returned to Idaho for the next year, I did not give this a second thought until moving back to Sayulita, Mexico in the fall of 2004. I had the opportunity to crew in a couple of informal fun races for the cruisers in the area. During conversations with several cruisers the topic of me being a yoga instructor came up, along with comments such as, "I would love to start yoga, but have no room on the boat" or, "I bought an Intro to Yoga book, but I have no place to lay a mat".

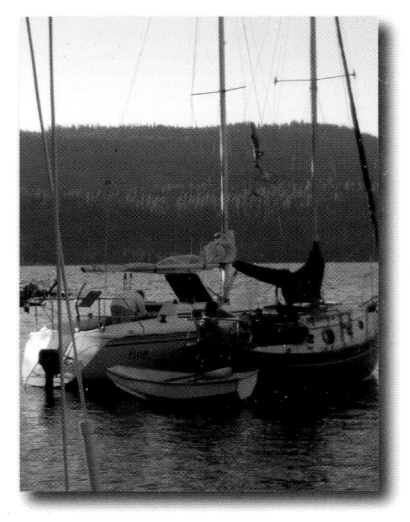

A seed had been planted.

Yoga Onboard is a guide that offers creative alternatives to the traditional approach to yoga postures and the encouragement to tap into one's own creativity to expand a practice beyond what I offer. Included in this guide is some very basic information about yoga as a whole, however, my intention is to offer a supplement to the many wonderful books on yoga that are already available: a supplement specifically for cruisers and live-aboards or others who may find themselves with limited space and a desire to continue their asana practice.

I love sailing. I love yoga. And I love sharing what I learn with others.
The opportunity to bring these together is an opportunity of a lifetime.

What is Yoga?

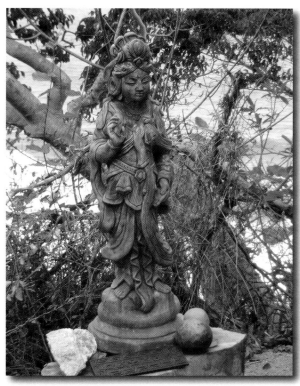

Yoga is an ancient body of knowledge dating back more than 7000 years. The word 'yoga' is brought to us from the sanskrit language and means 'to yoke' or 'union'. The yoga system is designed to bring us into union with our higher power. There are several paths that may be followed leading to this unity. *(see page 11)* The focus of Yoga Onboard is to use physical postures or *asana* as the vehicle to bring together the body, mind and spirit. Yoga is not a religion; however, it can be integrated into any religion or belief system seamlessly.

Looking back at the history of yoga, we can observe 4 distinct periods:

The *Vedic Period* brought us the Vedas, a collection of hymns which praise the divine power.

During the *Pre-Classical Period,* the Upanishads were created. These are 200 scriptures describing Brahma (a higher power), Atman (the self) and the relationship between the two.

The *Classical Period* is marked by the systemization of yoga by Pantanjali into what is known as the Yoga Sutras. It is through the Yoga Sutras that the concept of utilizing the body as a means to enlightenment was revitalized.

The focus of yoga shifts somewhat during the *Post-Classical Period* into more of a focus on the present, no longer striving to liberate us from reality, but teaching us acceptance and to live in the moment.

Yoga Sutras

Yoga is one of six systems of Indian philosophy outlined by the Yoga Sutras. The Yoga Sutras are the knowledge of yoga systemized and scripted by Patanjali, who is known as the Father of Yoga. They include everything necessary for the study and practice of yoga.

The eight Yoga Sutras are:
1. *Yamas* – abstinence or the "no's" of life
   a. *Ahimsa* – non-violence
   b. *Satya* – non-lying or seeking of truthfulness
   c. *Asteya* – non-stealing
   d. *Brahmacharya* – giving reverence through self restraint and moderation in sexual matters
   e. *Aparigraha* – non-hoarding
2. *Niyamas* – observances or the "yes's" of life
   a. *Saucha* – purity
   b. *Samtosha* – contentment
   c. *Tapas* – acceptance
   d. *Svadhyaya* – spiritual study
   e. *Isvara pranidhana* – life of dedication
3. *Asana* – posture achieving the following: alertness, grace, stability, comfort, steadiness and relaxation
4. *Pranayama* – breath control
5. *Pratyahara* - sense control or bringing the senses inside
6. *Dharana* – concentration
7. *Dhyana* – meditation
8. *Samadhi* – contemplation, absorption or super conscious state, oneness

Branches of Yoga

Yoga has six branches, each representing a particular approach to life. Like the tree, each branch is just as important as the others and each is a part of the whole. Practice in one of these paths does not preclude involvement in the others. Many times they naturally overlap.

Hatha Yoga is the yoga of postures, or physical practice. Yoga Onboard's focus lies within this path. We will focus on the physical poses as a vehicle toward unity.

Bhakti Yoga is the yoga of devotion. Expression of the devotional nature of every thought, word, and deed whether scrubbing the head or dealing with an angry neighbor is the primary focus here. Mahatma Gandhi, Martin Luther King, Jr. and Mother Teresa are all examples of Bhakti Yogis.

Raja Yoga is the yoga of self control. This path is based on the teachings of the Yoga Sutras. Raja means 'royal' and is considered to be the King of Yoga, because it constitutes a 'royal road' to happiness and fulfillment through meditation.

Jhana Yoga is the yoga of knowledge. Development of the intellect through the study of scriptures is the focus of this path.

Tantra Yoga is the yoga of rituals. The emphasis in tantra yoga is experiencing the Divine in everything. Through this an attitude of gratitude is cultivated, encouraging a ritualistic approach to life. Rituals associated with any rite of passage, including birthdays, anniversaries and holidays can create the reverent feelings that stem from tantra yoga.

Karma Yoga is the yoga of action or service. The principles of karma apply here and no one can escape this path. Karma is the belief that all of our present experiences are based on our past actions allowing us to consciously create a future of abundance and love. By engaging in selfless acts through donating our time, energy or money we can create a life that reflects our past actions.

Bring intention into your everyday.

Any movement, body position or activity can become part of your yoga practice, simply through intention. An intention guides your planned actions. Take, for instance, the activity of scrubbing the deck. Begin by noticing how your body is positioned. Are you on your hands and knees? Is your spine straight? If not, what could you do to align it? A simple repositioning of the knees under the hips can do wonders for how your back will feel afterward. Maybe your neck is strained. Make a conscious choice to relax the neck as the shoulder, arm and hand make circular motions. Even if we are exerting pressure in order to ensure a clean deck, we can find a place of relaxation. By focusing on the breath and the patterns of the cleanser this chore becomes a time of meditation. Just by doing these simple things you have practiced yoga. You have brought an awareness of the body and the breath into the mind. Building awareness is the first step in the process of bringing union into your life.

Yoga principles can be applied anywhere, anytime by anybody. Adapting traditional yoga postures to your space simply takes intention. Think about what your desired result is (relieving low back pressure – many times caused by tight hamstrings), determine what action is necessary to achieve your desired result (what postures can be practiced that will lengthen the hamstrings?), determine a place where you can practice these postures (in this case, the possibilities are endless!), then practice! We use the physical postures as a vehicle for examination with results becoming apparent in the strength and flexibility of the body, calmness within our selves as well as a feeling of connection. Just because there is not a flat open space or you don't have a yoga mat, does not mean that you cannot bring intention into your every day and experience the results of a daily yoga practice.

"To succeed you have to believe in something with such passion that it becomes a reality."

Anita Roddick

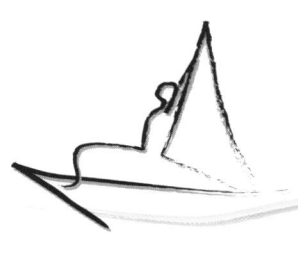

Remember to...

ॐ Begin your practice with a few minutes of meditation.

ॐ Move with mindfulness.

ॐ Create space in the body by lengthening the spine
and lifting the heart center.

ॐ Your body is your teacher. Listen to it.

ॐ Use the breath as your guide.

ॐ Ideally try to choose the same time each day to practice.

Designing your practice

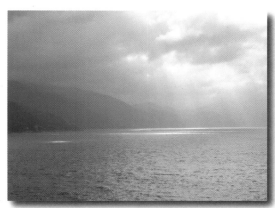

Approach each *asana* as you would approach your sailing. When going for a sail you never just raise the sails, point the boat in the direction you want to go and expect to arrive at your destination. There are external factors such as wind direction and speed as well as currents to consider, and don't forget internal factors such as the make and size of the boat or how much extra weight is being carried. All of this determines the fine tuning that takes place, the points of sail that need to be taken in order to get from point A to point B. When moving into an *asana*, take your time, feel your way into it. Then after a couple of breaths, listen - fine tune - adjust your sails. Let the breath guide you deeper, just as the wind takes you across the water.

Once you have felt your way into a pose, hold for 3-5 breaths or longer if it feels good. Each breath should be long and relaxed, approximately a 3-4 count for each inhale and each exhale. By breathing through the nose, we hold the heat within the body and calm the mind. Find a place within the pose where you are working, but comfortable.

Most of all, remember to have fun!

Think of your body and your boat as a playground and you are a child
                                        ...explore   what feels good? what doesn't?

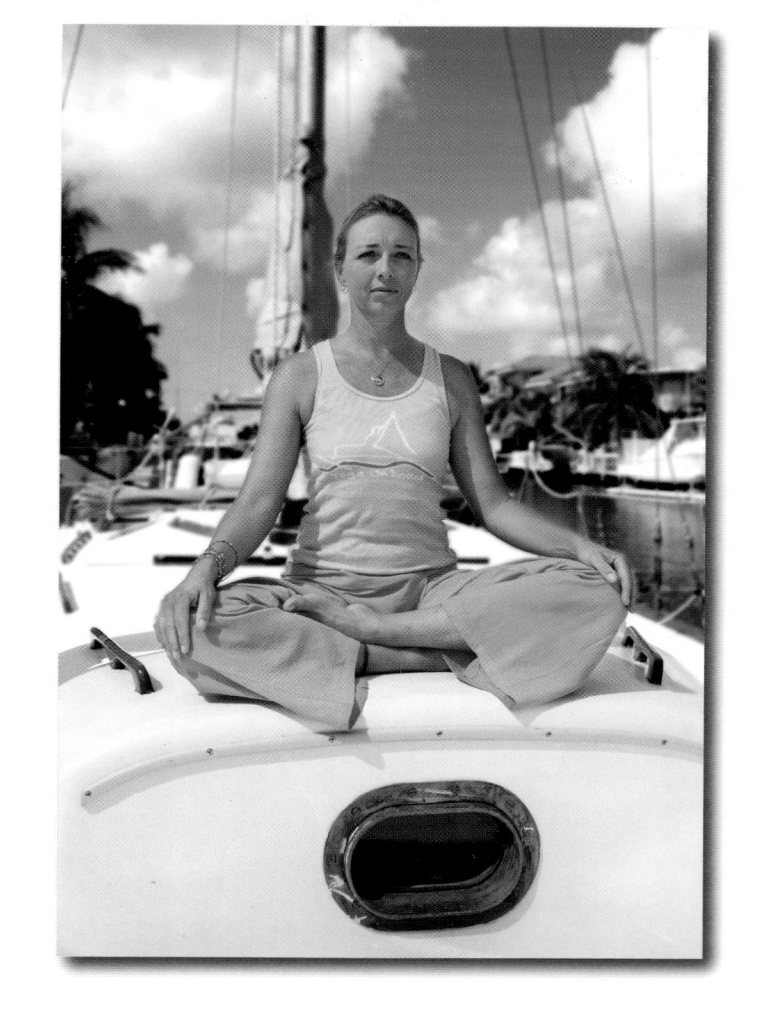

Pay attention to the breath. Think about the breath. When we are thinking about the breath, our mind is focused on one thing—this is concentration. Through concentration we find meditation.

Notice each inhale.   *Notice each exhale.*

Notice the space between the inhales and exhales, and the exhales and the inhales.

Hear the breath.   *See the breath.*
Feel the breath.   *Taste the breath.*

The more we breathe consciously, the stiller our mind becomes, and the more peaceful we feel.

It is said that the breath is the bridge between the material world and the spiritual world. By bringing attention to our breath we invite spirit into our bodies. *Pranayama* is made up of two words, *prana* which means life force and *yama* which means to restrain or control. Bringing the life force into our physical bodies consciously allows us to begin the process of unity.

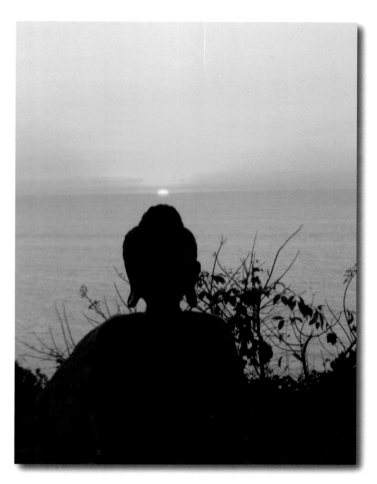

This doesn't have to be difficult or elusive. Meditation is simply a matter of concentrating on one thing for an extended period - even if you begin with only a few minutes.

Simply sit in a comfortable position and breathe. Focus on each breath, how the body feels, the thoughts that are running through your head (and they will, trust me) as a neutral observer, just notice, always coming back to the breath. Make it simple, make it easy. You can focus on the breath with your eyes closed, watch the designs in the water, or the clouds drift across the sky. Notice any movements of the boat. Are you in a calm anchorage? Is there a small swell gently rocking the boat? Think about how you will incorporate these into your practice. Whatever happens is perfect.

Being a sailor, I am guessing you have meditated many times. It is simply a matter of bringing awareness to the times you sit and stare at the water for an indefinite amount of time as the wind and the auto pilot work their magic. How many sunsets have you watched without thinking of anything but that big orange ball lowering itself toward the horizon?

"Tell me what you pay attention to and
I will tell you who you are."
Jose Ortega Gasset

The Postures
asana

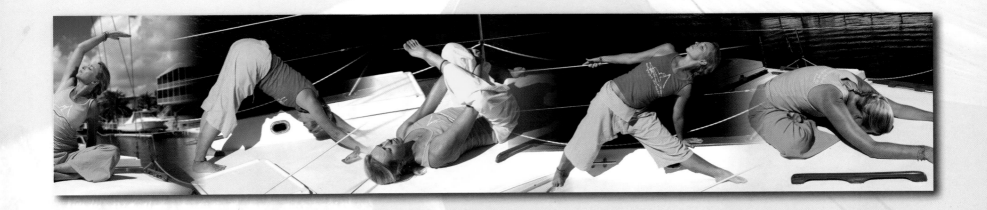

This is a short series of easy stretches that are great to do upon awakening or anytime throughout the day.

Easily adapt this sequence to the cockpit for a quick pick me up during a long night watch. Simply begin with the bottoms of your feet firmly planted on the sole of the cockpit, making sure your body is in complete alignment.

Begin in a comfortable cross-legged position, easy pose or *sukasana*. As with any pose, hold each of these poses for 3-5 breaths or longer if it feels good.

Neck Rolls: Drop the chin to the chest then gently make a few big circles with the head, first one direction, then the other. Pay attention to how the rest of the body responds to this movement.

1. Walk your hands out in front of you, releasing your head toward the deck. For balance, switch how your legs are crossed and repeat.

2. Press your hands behind you as you lift your heart and your chin. Breathe and feel the entire front of the body open.

listen

3. Use one arm for support as you lift and reach the other over the head, stretching the side of the torso. Switch sides.

4. Place a hand on the opposite knee. Using the breath, inhale and grow taller, exhale and look over the shoulder, twisting the torso and stimulating the spine. Switch sides.

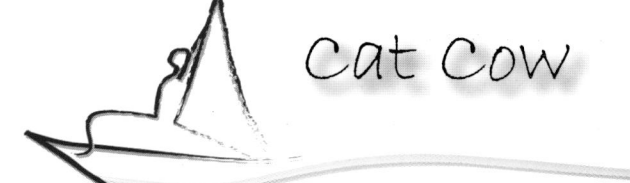

Cat Cow

Come to your hands and knees—wrists below shoulders, knees below hips, with a neutral spine

1. Connect with your breath.

2. Inhale — lift the chin and sit bones, dropping the belly (cow pose).

3. Exhale — tuck the chin and tailbone, rounding the back (cat pose).

4. Repeat 3-5 times.

be mindful

Benefits:
Opens the front and back of the torso, stimulates the spine and builds awareness of the connection between breath and movement. Also feels great after backbends!

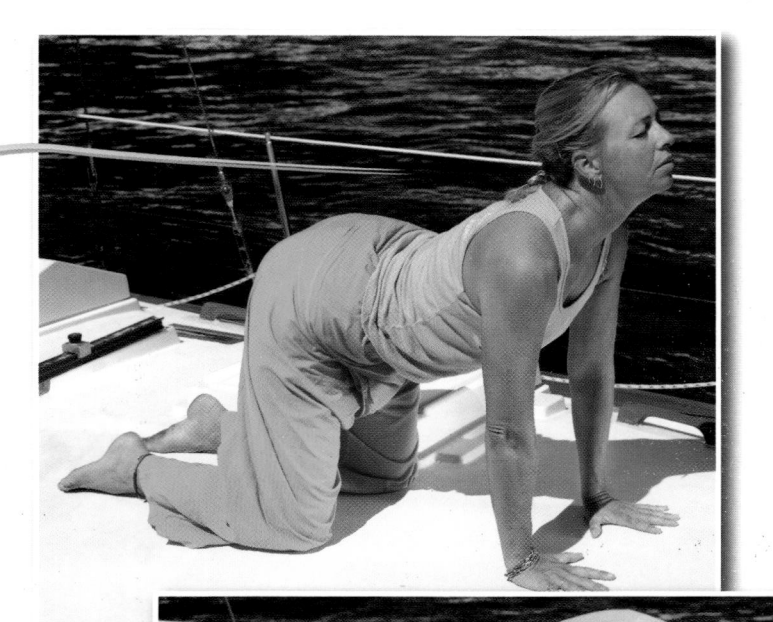

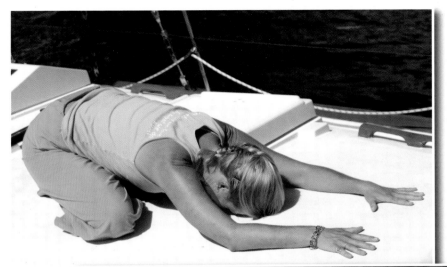

Child's Pose
balasana

This is a great resting pose that can be done between more challenging asana.

Begin on your hands and knees.

1. Widen your knees just enough to rest the torso gently between your thighs.

2. Place your sit bones on your heels, resting your forehead on the deck.

3. Rest your hands either back by your feet or extended.
   Again, what feels good?

4. Completely relax.

listen

Benefits:
Releases stress, increases circulation to the brain, elongates the back and spine and gently stretches the hips, thighs and ankles.

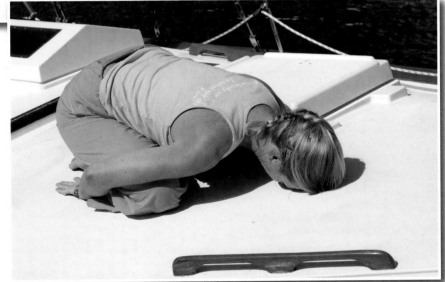

"I do this all the time, at random intervals during the day when I am stressed. It does so much for me." Melanie Neale

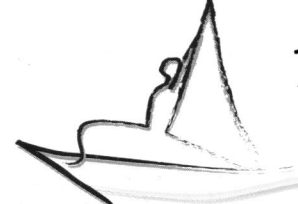

Downward Facing Dog
adho muka svanasana

1. From your hands and knees, tuck your toes under.

2. On the exhale, press into hands with the fingers spread wide, lifting sit bones upward.

3. Draw the shoulders toward the thighs forming an inverted V.

4. Relax your head downward.

5. Feet should be hip distance apart and hands shoulder distance apart, with big toes and middle finger facing forward.

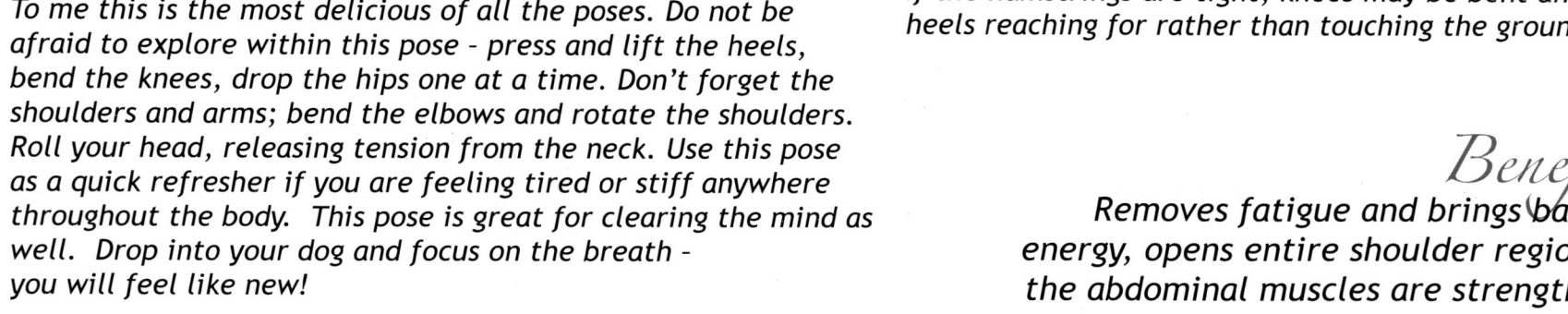

If the hamstrings are tight, knees may be bent and heels reaching for rather than touching the ground.

To me this is the most delicious of all the poses. Do not be afraid to explore within this pose – press and lift the heels, bend the knees, drop the hips one at a time. Don't forget the shoulders and arms; bend the elbows and rotate the shoulders. Roll your head, releasing tension from the neck. Use this pose as a quick refresher if you are feeling tired or stiff anywhere throughout the body. This pose is great for clearing the mind as well. Drop into your dog and focus on the breath – you will feel like new!

Benefits:
Removes fatigue and brings back lost energy, opens entire shoulder region, and the abdominal muscles are strengthened.

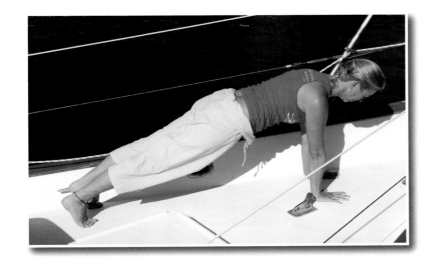

Plank Pose

1. Place wrists directly below your shoulders.

2. Look slightly ahead of you keeping the entire spine long.

3. Reach the heels back as you engage the entire core of the body.

To modify this pose for beginners or persons with less strength in their core, drop the knees to the ground, keeping the back straight.

Four Limbed Staff Pose
chataranga dandasana

1. Begin in plank pose. Continue to engage the core.

2. Keeping the elbows in tight to the body and the eyes forward, lower down until you are hovering over the ground. (You may need to slide the body forward so the elbows are over the wrists)

To modify this pose, begin with knees down, then drop the chest and chin between the hands.

These two poses are used as part of a flow in the sun salutations. (see pages 63-65)

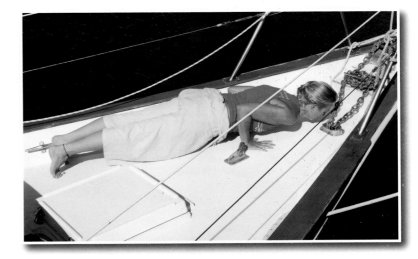

Benefits:
Tones and strengthens entire core, shoulders to hips.

25

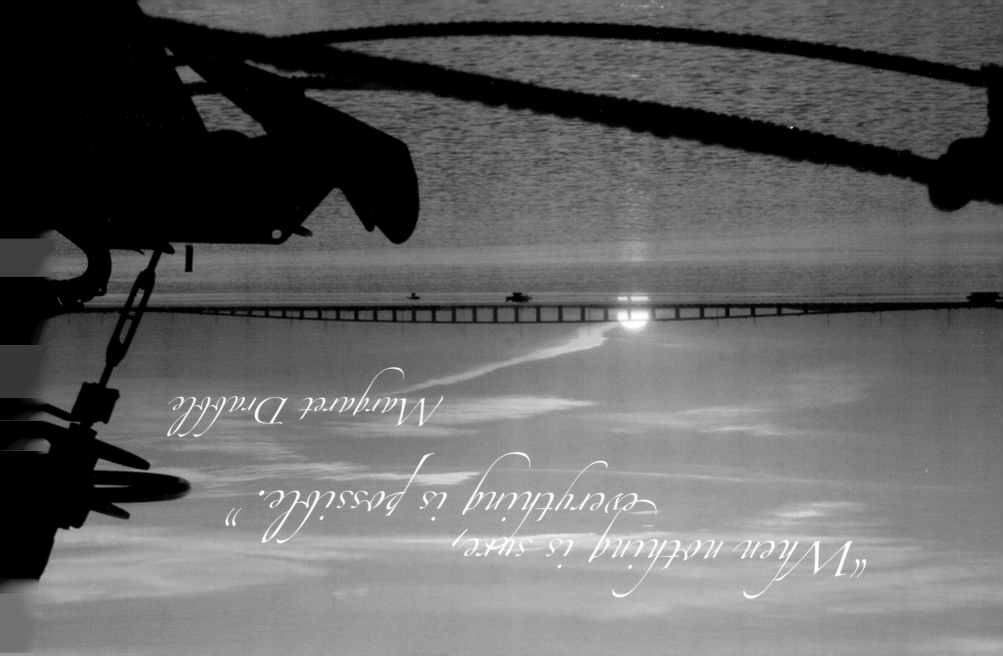

"When nothing is sure, everything is possible."

Margaret Drabble

standing Poses

We use standing postures to increase stength in the leg muscles and joints and to increase the blood supply to this area, preventing circulation problems within the lower limbs.

On a boat, many standing postures also become balancing postures depending on the weather or heel at the time of your practice. Use this as an opportunity to build awareness as to how the body reacts to the movement. We are accustomed to moving with the boat, but are we really aware of what is happening within ourselves?

Mountain Pose
Extended Mountain Pose
Standing Forward Fold
Tree Pose
Triangle Pose
Warrior I
Warrior II
Warrior III
Heart & Back Openers
Standing Twist

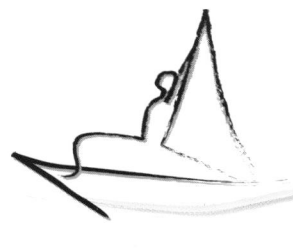

Mountain Pose
tadasana

1. Begin by standing with the feet hip-distance apart with equal pressure on all four corners of the feet. The toes are relaxed.

2. Lift your knee caps, engaging the upper legs.

3. Tuck the tailbone just slightly, lift the heart center and reach the top of the head upward, lengthening the entire spine.

4. Allow your shoulders to relax back and down; relax your facial muscles.

5. The arms are extended down at the sides.

breathe

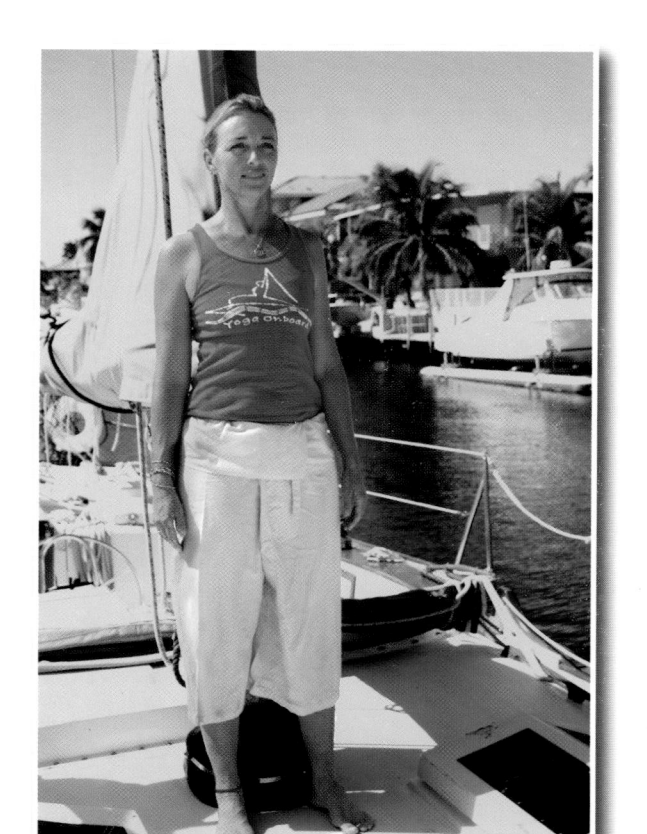

This is the foundation for all of our standing postures. Do not underestimate the power of this seemingly still pose.

Extended Mountain Pose
utthita tadasana

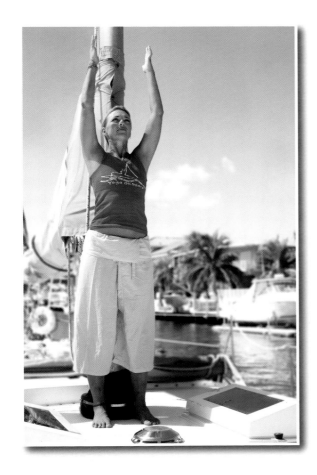

Benefits:

Both mountain pose and extended mountain pose tone the leg muscles and give one a sense of balance and poise.

1. Begin in mountain pose, inhale and extend your arms above your head.

2. Lower and relax your shoulders.

be mindful

"Each asana and each breath is a complete journey."
David Swenson

Standing Forward Fold
uttanasana

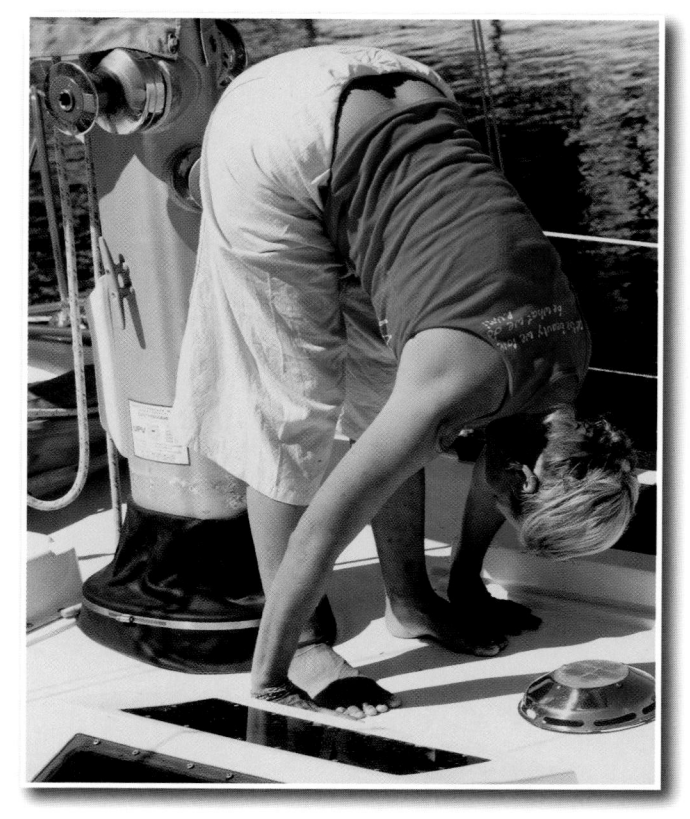

1. Begin in mountain pose or extended mountain pose.

2. On the exhale, bend forward from the hips, keeping your spine straight. Bend your knees, if necessary, to protect the lower back.

During forward folds keep the back straight and move from the hips. Never bend from the waist. This will round the back and create strain in the lower back.

listen

Benefits:
Massages the stomach, helps depression, tones the liver and lengthens the hamstrings.

Standing Forward Fold Variation

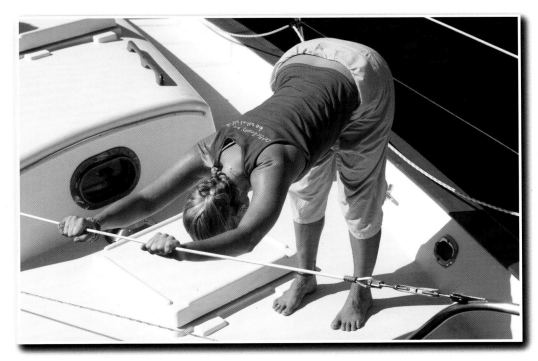

1. Position yourself far enough away from the lifelines to enable you to extend your arms fully with your hips over your ankles.

2. Firmly plant your feet and lift the kneecaps, engaging the upper thighs.

3. Use the lifeline for support to keep the spine long. Hold your head in a comfortable position.

4. If you feel any pressure in the low back, bend your knees.

Using the lifelines in this manner allows you to safely begin lengthening the hamstrings and opening the shoulders and upper arms.

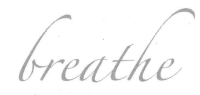

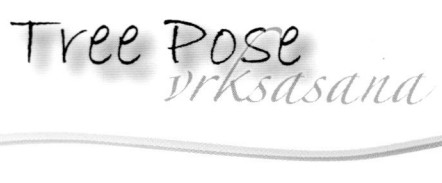

Tree Pose
vrksasana

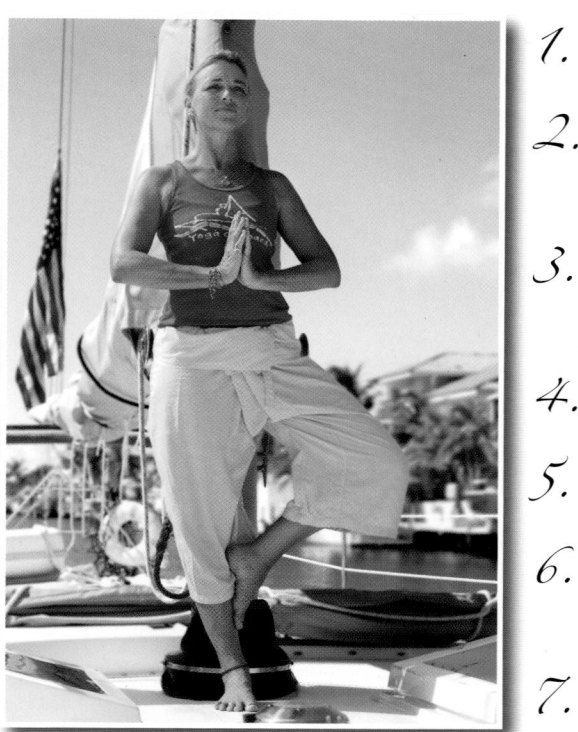

1. Begin in mountain pose.

2. Bring one foot to the ankle, calf, or inner thigh— avoid the knee area.

3. Lengthen through the center of the body.

4. Bring the hands to prayer.

5. Breathe - then extend arms upward.

6. Use the mast for alignment and support.

7. Switch sides.

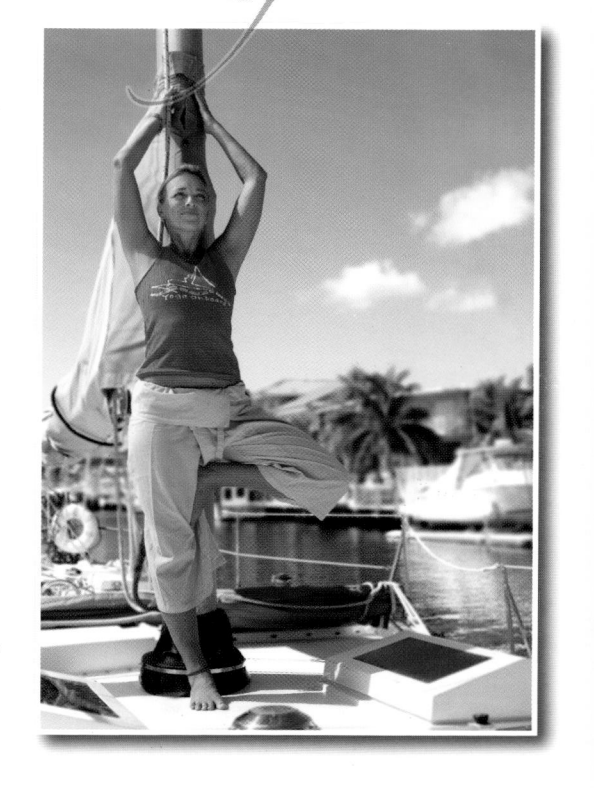

Benefits:
Tones the leg muscles and gives one a sense of balance and poise.

Triangle Pose
utthita trikonasana

1. Begin with your legs wide, your left foot facing to the left, the right foot facing straight.

2. Extend your arms out to the sides and relax your shoulders.

3. Slide your body to the left, lower the upper body from the hips; keeping your shoulders in alignment with the legs.

4. Lower your left hand to the deck or your shin.

5. Either use the lifeline for support or extend the right arm upward, looking up.

6. Keep both knees active.

7. Switch sides

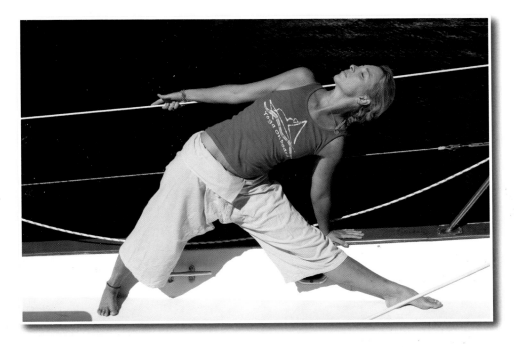

listen

Benefits:
Tones the legs, relieves back aches and strengthens the ankles.

warrior I
virabhadrasana I

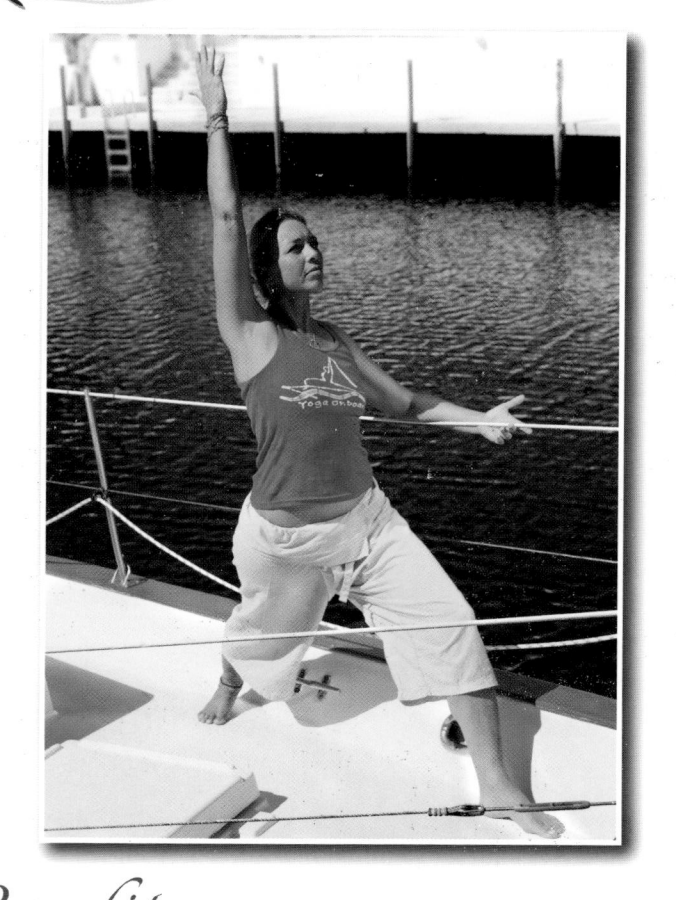

1. Begin in mountain pose. Step your right foot back.

2. Both feet are flat with the front foot straight ahead and the back foot in a 45-60 angle.

3. Bend your front knee, keeping the knee over or behind your ankle, taking the feet wider if necessary to allow the hips to lower adding strength to the pose.

4. Both hips are facing forward, your heart is lifting and the shoulders are relaxed.

5. Your arms can be on the hips, extended upward or using the lifelines for support.

6. Switch sides.

breathe

Benefits:
Relieves stiffness in shoulders and back, tones the legs and reduces fat around hips.

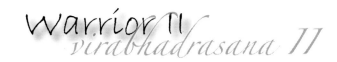

Warrior II
virabhadrasana II

Moving from warrior I into warrior II is a natural transition.

1. From warrior I, open your hips and shoulders to face the side.

2. The front knee stays bent, your back leg straight and strong.

3. Stretch your arms out to the sides. Imagine extending far enough to touch both ends of your boat, or utilize the life lines for support.

4. Eyes are gazing softly forward over the front shoulder.

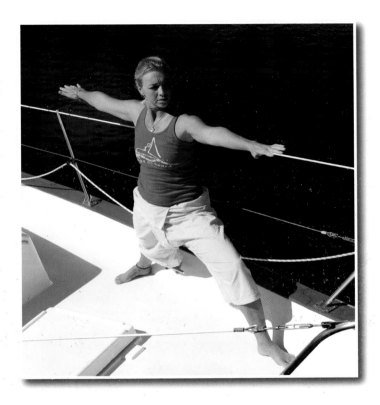

Benefits:
The leg muscles become stronger and more elastic, preparing for lengthening of the hamstrings; also tones the abdominal organs.

The Story of Virabhadra

The warrior postures are dedicated to the powerful hero and great warrior, Virabhadra.

Daksha, the chief of the gods, made arrangements for a huge celebration and didn't invite his daughter Sati's husband Shiva, the Supreme God. Sati, although deeply insulted, attended the celebration. Distraught with humiliation, she threw herself into the fire and perished. When Shiva heard this news, he burned with anger. Tearing from his head a lock of hair, glowing with energy, he threw it to the ground. Out of this sprang Virabhadra, tall enough to reach the high heavens, dark as the clouds with a thousand arms, three burning eyes and fiery hair. Virabhadra bowed at Shiva's feet and asked his will.

"Lead my army against Daksha and destroy his celebration.", ordered Shiva. Virabhadra proceeded to Daksha's assembly with Shiva's entire army with him, leaving nothing intact, finally cutting off the head of Daksha.

Virabhadra is prominently worshipped today in South India. The famous Lepakshi temple in Andhra Pradesh is dedicated to Lord Virabhadra.

Warrior III
virabhadrasana III

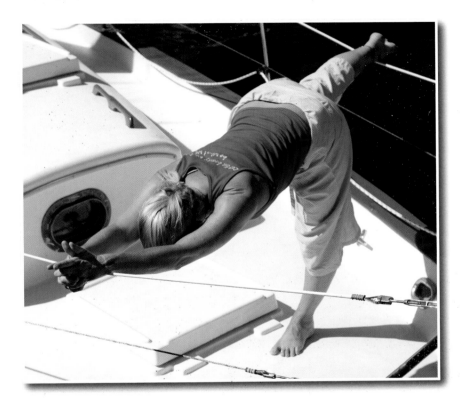

1. Begin by placing yourself in the variation for standing forward fold.

2. With your hands on the lifeline, keep the hips square, lift an extended leg up behind you. If your vessel allows it, you may place your foot on the opposite lifeline for added support.

3. While this is a balancing pose, it also uses the core of the body to maintain structure.

4. The extended leg and the arms are parallel to the deck.

5. Switch sides.

Benefits:
Tones the legs and abdominals as well as conveys poise, power and harmony with the body and mind.

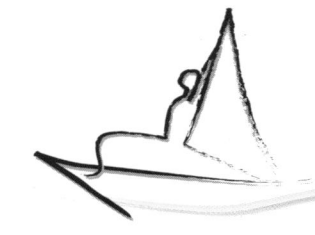

Heart and Back Openers

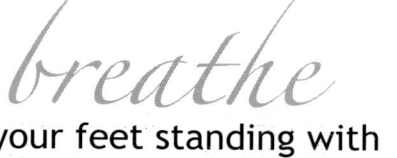
breathe

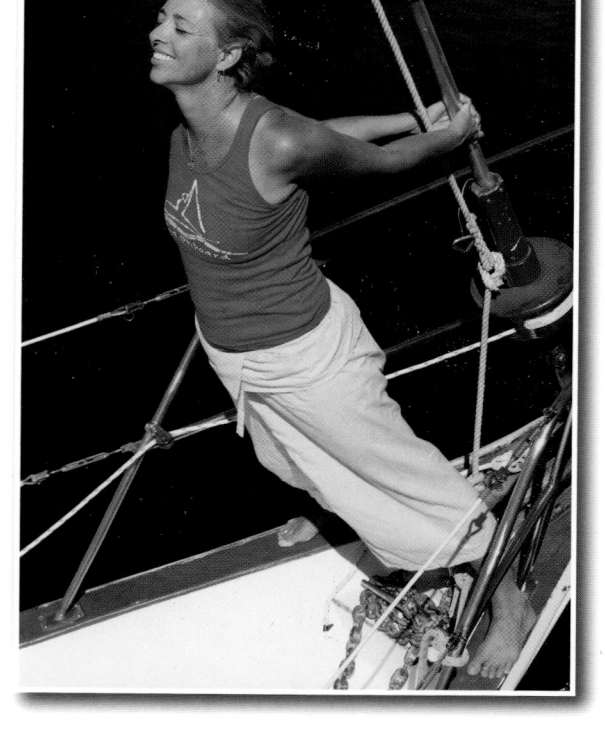

1. Begin by feeling the bottoms of your feet standing with equal pressure on all four corners.

2. Using the forestay as support, either open the heart center or round the back—tailbone to crown.

3. Tuck the tailbone and bend the knees slightly for balance in both poses.

Be conscious of the part of the body you are opening, and breathe into that area. Adjust the pose by moving your hands either higher or lower on the forestay, finding just the right stretch.

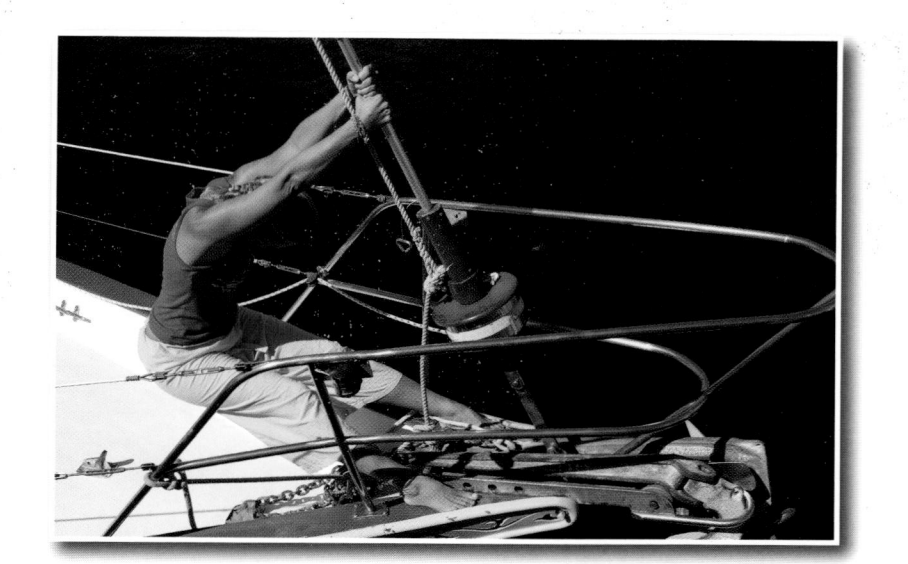

be mindful

1. Set your foundation: equal standing on both feet, facing away from the forestay.

2. Stabilize your hips using one hand, in order to protect the low back.

3. Use the forestay to assist balance and to deepen your twist.

4. Look over your shoulder, using the breath to lengthen the spine.

Remember, where the eyes go, the body will follow. This truth can also be applied to life as well. When we hold onto a clear vision of what it is we desire, it naturally follows that we will achieve.

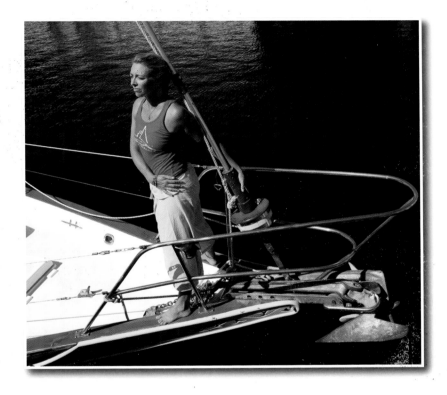

Benefits:

All twists stretch and open the torso, aid in keeping the digestive system healthy and stimulate the spine.

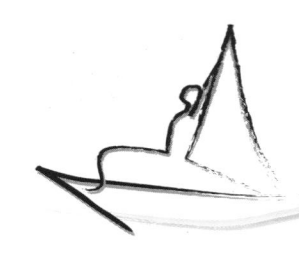

A Word on Transitions

In my classes I teach a vinyasa flow class. What this means is that with each breath a movement is linked. There is a natural flow from one posture to the next. When practicing on the boat, sometimes you will find yourself moving from one area of the boat to another. Maybe your standing postures are on the bow and your forward folds are in the cockpit. Wherever you decide each pose works best for you, move from one to another with purpose. By holding your intention even as you walk from one end of the boat to another, your practice is uninterrupted. As we have all heard many times, it is about the journey. It is about remaining present and focused on the now while maintaining a vision of the future. Even as you transition from posture to posture be conscious and mindful.

"It is good to have an end to journey toward; but it is the journey that matters in the end"
Ursula K. LeGuin

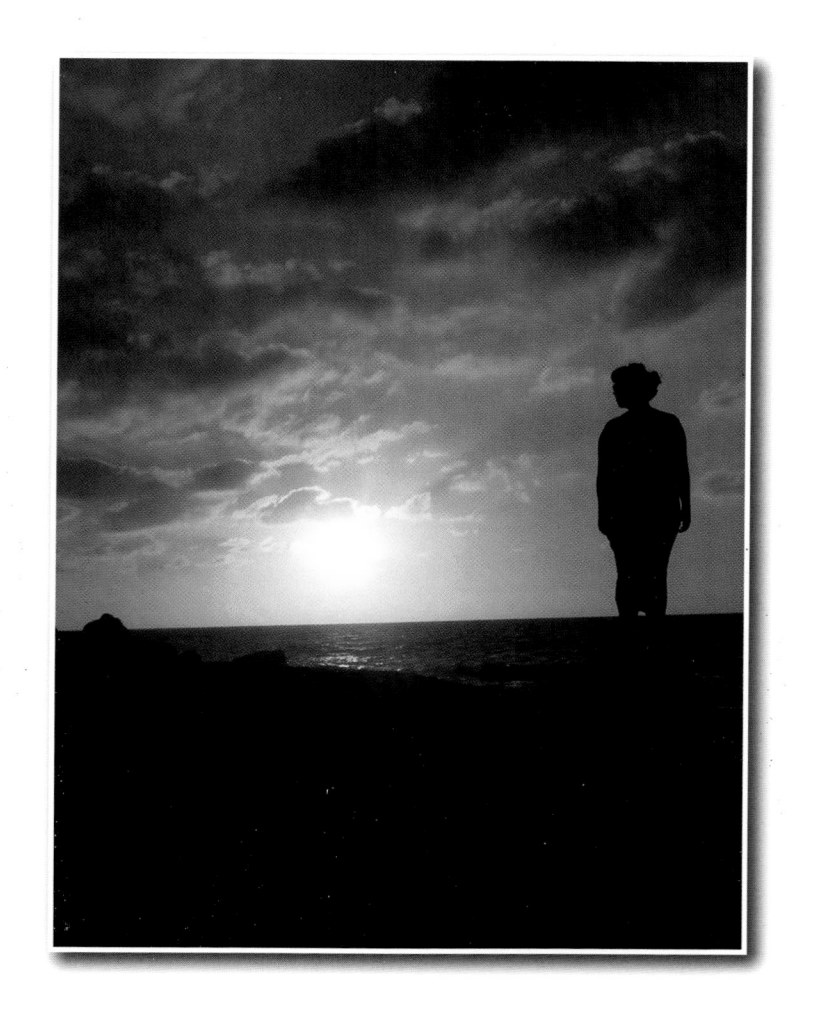

Backbends

Most of the time our daily activities call for our arms to be reaching or working in front of the body causing the shoulders to slouch, the muscles in the chest to shorten and the heart center to close. Through the practice of backbends we create the opportunity to reverse the effects of this. Backbends offer us the opportunity to symbolically open ourselves to the future by physically opening the front of the body.

Benefits:

With all backbends the central nervous system is stimulated increasing the ability to deal with stress. Through stimulation of the spine and an opening of the heart, relief for headaches and hypertension is found. The back muscles are strengthened and the abdominals are toned. Backbends are invaluable for sufferers of depression. Just the simple act of physically opening the heart center gives one a sense of joy.

Cobra
Sphinx Pose
Upward Facing Dog

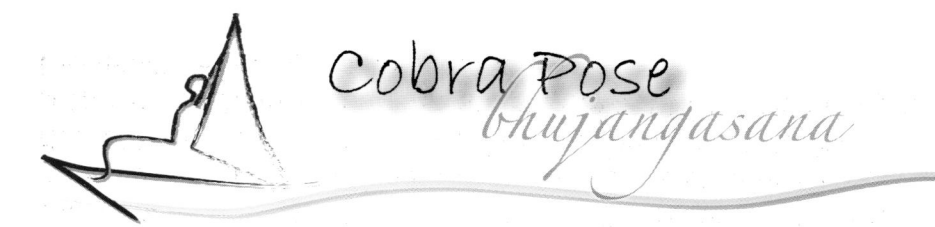

cobra pose
bhujangasana

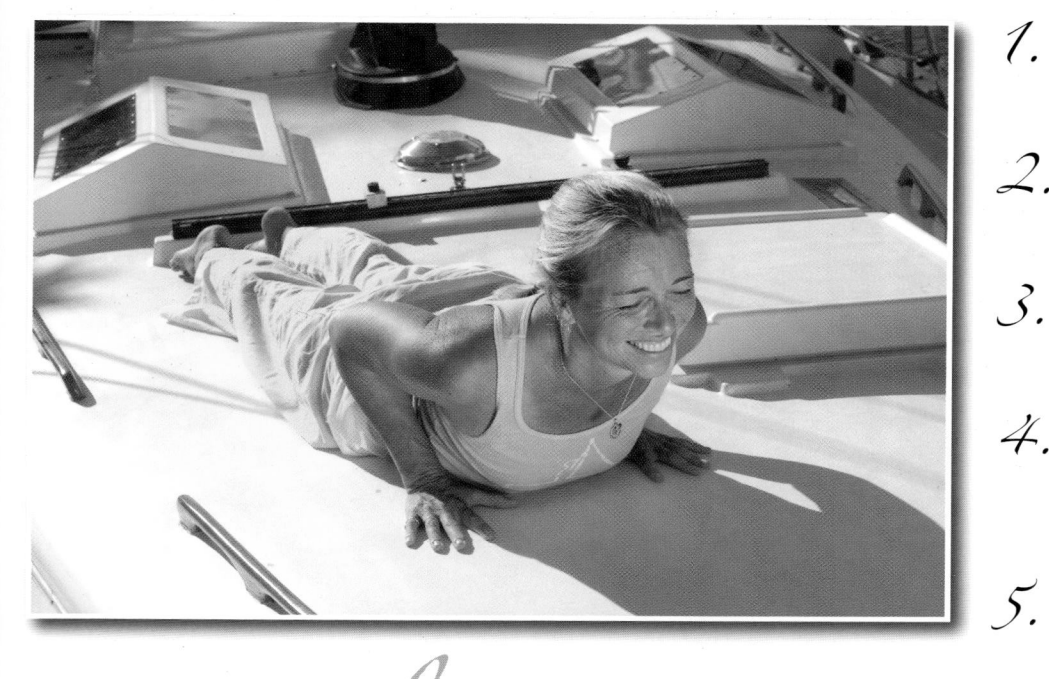

listen

1. Begin on your belly with your legs and feet coming together like a long cobra tail.

2. Place your hands under the shoulders, with your thumbs touching the rib cage.

3. Reach the elbows towards one another, bringing the shoulder blades together.

4. At the same time, reach the elbows toward your heels, allowing your heart to lift and reach forward.

5. Eyes can be straight ahead or slightly elevated—what feels good?

6. Relax and breathe into the back.

This pose can be taken deeper by pressing into the hands, allowing the heart to lift upward.

Sphinx Pose

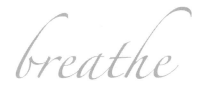

1. Begin on your belly with your elbows directly under the shoulders. Your palms are flat.

2. Tuck your tailbone, lengthening the lower spine.

3. Press into your elbows, creating length in the spine and space in the torso.

4. Reach your heart forward as you bring your shoulder blades together.

5. Eyes are looking straight ahead. Imagine the sphinx statues in Egypt.

6. Relax the neck and facial muscles.

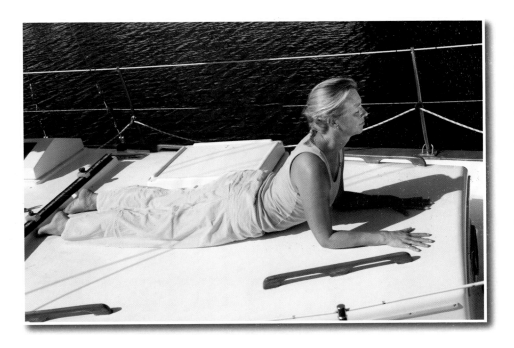

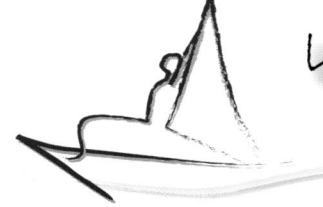

upward Facing Dog
urdva muka svanasana

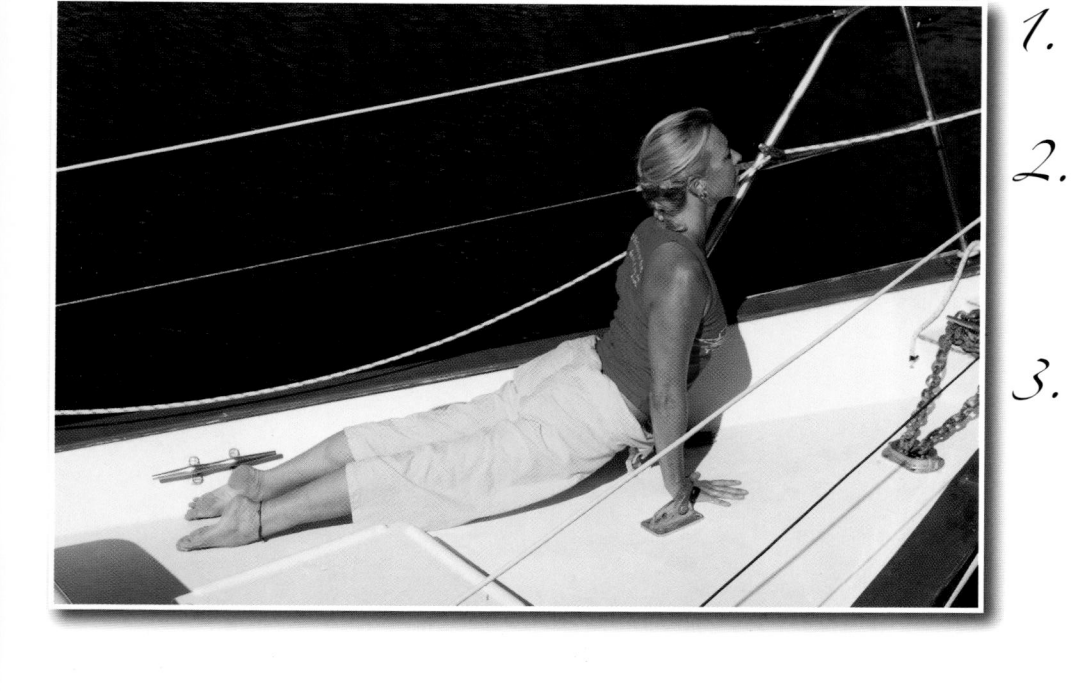

1. From your belly, place your hands next to the center of the rib cage.

2. Press into your hands as you roll your shoulders back and lift the heart upwards. Your hands will be directly below your shoulders.

3. Allow your eyes to gaze softly upward, keeping the neck long.

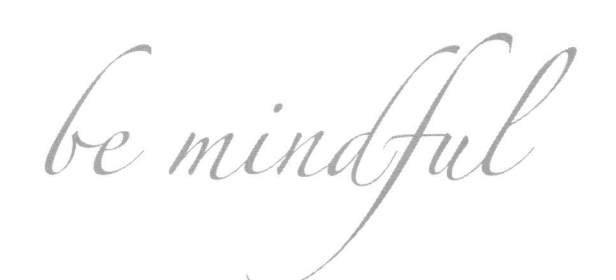

To strengthen this pose, *press firmly into the tops of the feet and lift the knees and thighs off the ground. Engage the core of the body by pulling the belly button in to protect the low back.*

Seated Poses

Our seated postures include our foundation pose, forward folds, hip openers and an abdominal strengthener. They are best done after a complete cycle of standing postures to ensure that the muscles are warm and ready to be lengthened. With all seated postures, begin with the sit bones connecting evenly, the spine straight and the legs active. It is important to remain energetic and fully alert in each posture. All seated postures bring a sense of peace and calmness to the mind and it is often easy to become careless or laid-back once you are to this point in your practice. Take a deep invigorating breath and continue your practice with full awareness.

Staff Pose
Seated Forward Fold
Head to Knee Pose
Bound Angle Pose
Hip Openers
Supine Half Lotus Pose
Firelog Pose
Cow Face Pose
Boat Pose

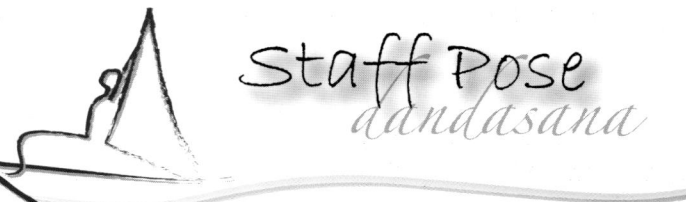

Staff Pose
dandasana

This is the foundation for all of our seated postures. This posture is exactly like mountain pose except for a 90 degree angle in the hips. Every muscle is active and participating, just as in our standing foundation. Again, do not underestimate the power of this seemingly simple pose.

listen

1. Extend your legs in front of you.

2. The feet are flat just as if you were standing. Activate your leg muscles.

3. Your shoulders are over the hips and relaxed with your heart lifting upward.

4. The top of your head is reaching upward and the eyes are gazing directly ahead.

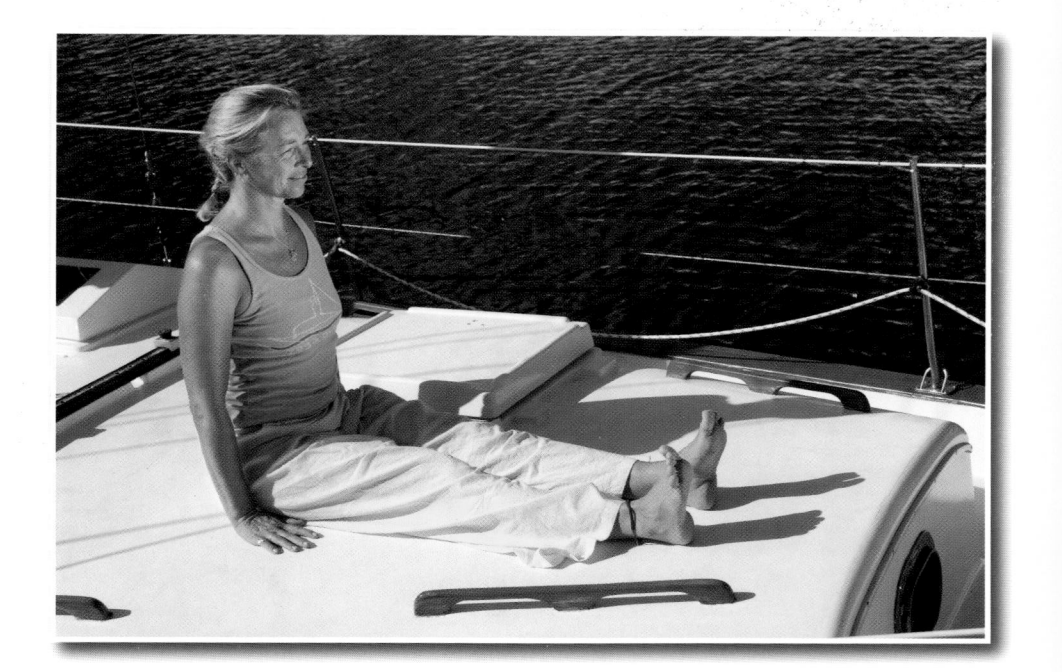

Benefits:
Builds awareness of posture and can be used for meditation.

Seated Forward Fold
paschimottanasana

1. Begin in staff pose. Focus on keeping the back straight and long, pull your shoulders back and open the heart center.

2. Slowly begin to reach your heart toward the feet, keeping your eyes focused just beyond the tips of the toes.

3. As your flexibility increases and your belly reaches your thighs, your head can rest gently onto your knees or shins. Reach the elbows outward allowing the heart to remain open.

breathe

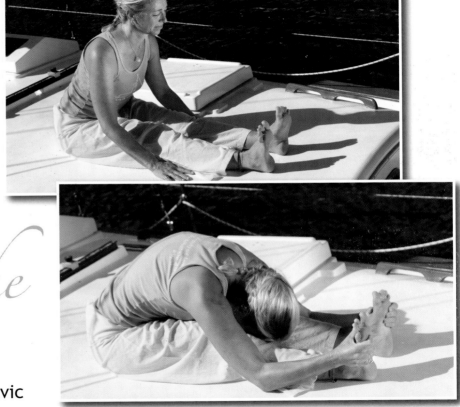

Benefits:
Increases flexibility in the hamstrings and strengthens the back, increases circulation to pelvic region and massages internal organs.

Remember, this pose is not about touching your toes, it is about lengthening the hamstrings and strengthening the back.

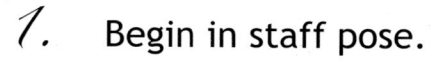

Head to Knee Pose
janu sirsasana

1. Begin in staff pose.

2. Bring your right foot to your inner left thigh.

3. Rotate your body so that it is square with the extended leg, keeping that leg active.

4. Reach your heart forward, moving from the hips.

5. Release your head towards your knee.

6. Switch sides.

be mindful

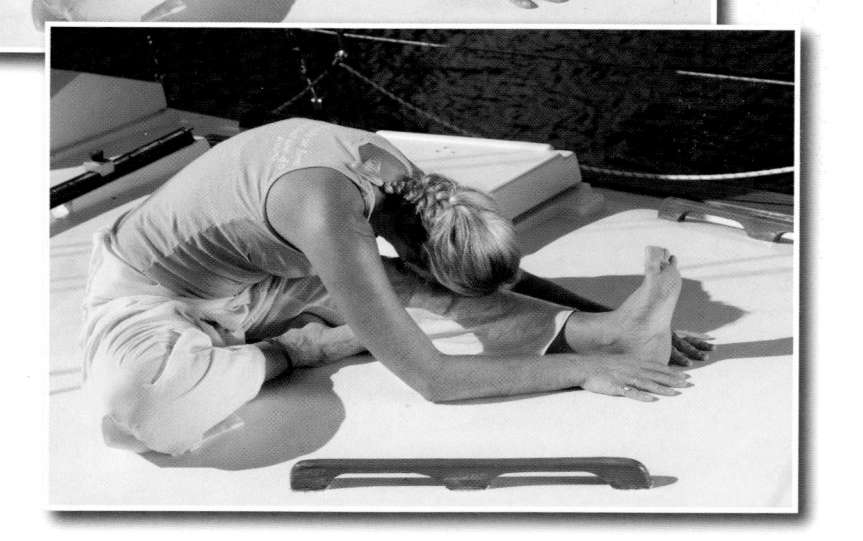

Benefits: Besides lengthening the hamstring, this posture aids digestion and tones and activates the kidneys.

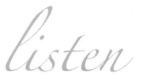

Staff Pose

Seated Forward Fold

Head to Knee Pose

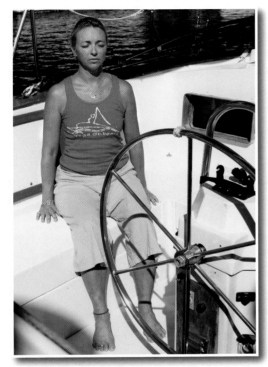

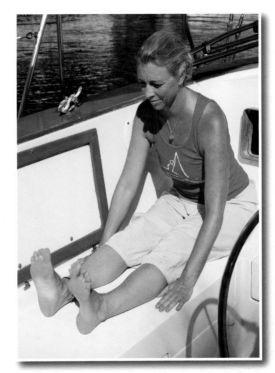

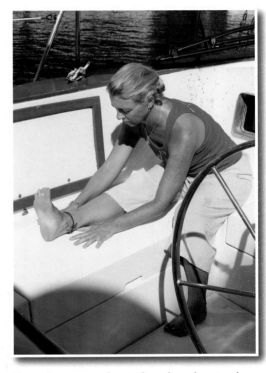

Merge your sit bones with the seat. Both feet are on the sole of the cockpit. Lengthen through the spine and breathe.

Bring both legs up onto the seat and continue with a traditional seated forward fold.

Keeping one foot firmly planted on the sole of the cockpit, extend and activate the opposite leg on the seat. Continue with a traditional head to knee pose.

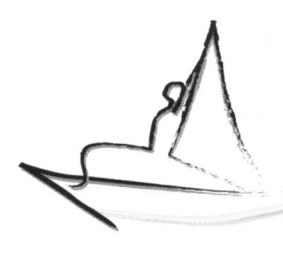

Using Sail Ties

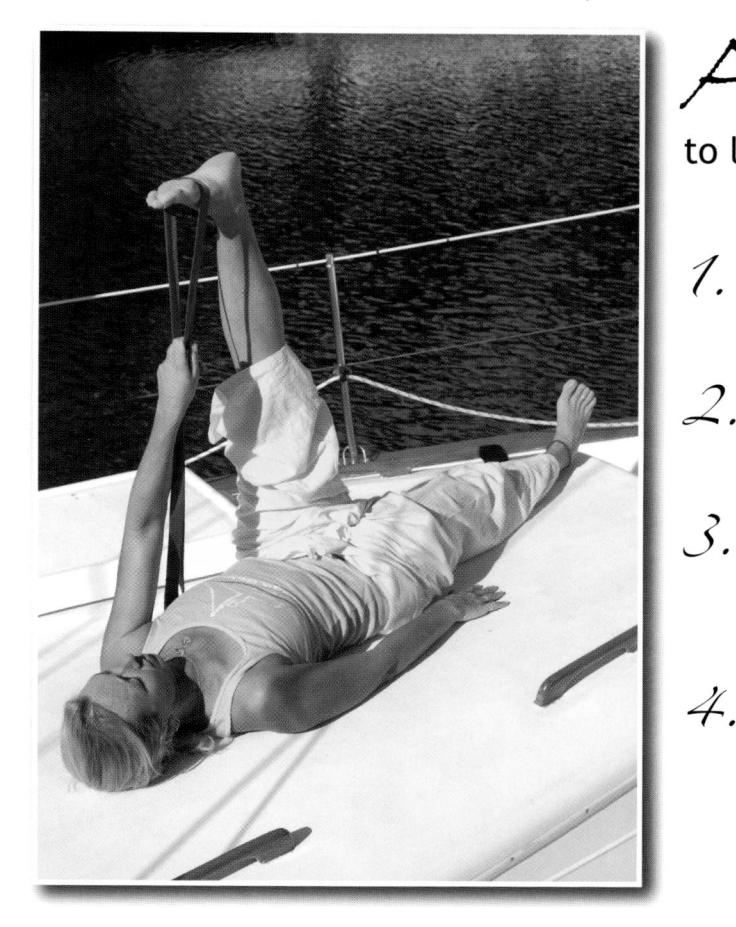

An alternative for lengthening the hamstrings for those that have lower back problems or extremely tight hamstrings is to lie on your back and work with one leg at a time.

1. Bring one leg up and place a sail tie around the flexed foot. Your knee may remain bent.

2. Using the sail tie to keep the leg extended, slowly begin to straighten the leg.

3. Once you have come to a point where the leg is straight (keep in mind, this may take months!) you can again use the sail tie to gently pull the leg towards you.

4. Switch sides.

breathe

1. Begin in staff pose.

2. Bring the bottoms of the feet together a comfortable distance from the hips, holding onto the feet or ankles.

3. Bring awareness into the spine, keeping it long and straight as you lift and reach the heart center forward.

be mindful

Benefits: This pose increases the circulation to the hips, abdomen, pelvis and back. It is great for any reproductive issues.

This pose is sometimes called Cobblers Pose after the cobblers in India who would hold their work between their feet.

Hip Openers

Good hip flexibility is essential in virtually all hatha yoga postures, from sitting in easy pose (*sukasana*) to most standing postures. This flexibility affects our forward folds, twists and meditative postures. The most basic of hip openers is to simply lie on your back and pull your knees toward your chest. Begin with the knees together for a few breaths then open the knees toward the armpits and breathe.

Supine Half Lotus

1. Begin on your back with your knees pulled into your chest.

2. Cross your right ankle over your left knee.

3. Reach between your legs with the right arm and grab onto your left shin or thigh.

4. Relax the shoulders and head.

5. Switch sides.

listen

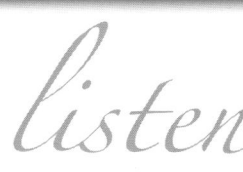

Firelog Pose

1. Begin in easy pose.

2. Cross your legs with the ankle over the knee and the knee over the ankle so the shins are lined up over one another.

3. Flex the feet and lengthen the spine by sitting up tall.

4. Switch sides.

breathe

"The Sea yeelds Action to the bodie,
Meditation to the Minde."
Samuel Purchas

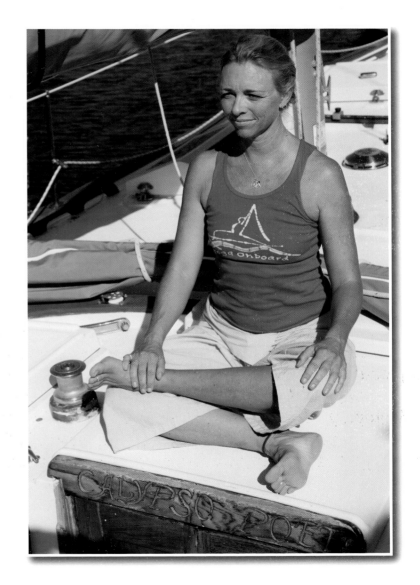

be mindful

1. Begin in easy pose *(sukasana)*.

2. Cross your legs with one knee over the other.

3. Connect both sit bones to the deck with your heels equal distance from your hips.

4. Lengthen through the spine.

5. Switch sides.

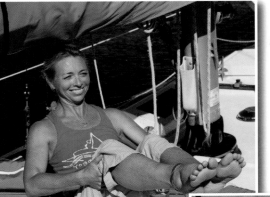

Begin with knees bent

Boat Pose
navasana

1. Begin in staff pose.

2. Raise your legs up, keeping the spine long and straight and balance on your sit bones.

3. Lift the heart center and bring your belly button in towards spine.

4. Relax your face and shoulders.

5. Hold for 5 breaths then release to resting position.

As your core strengthens, straighten your legs.

Resting position:
Toes and fingertips touch the ground lightly. Tuck the chin and tailbone, rounding the spine. See Yoga on s/v Spellbound, page 72.

Repeat this sequence 3-5 times.

Benefits:
Strengthens all core muscles including abdominals, back and psoas.

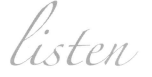

listen

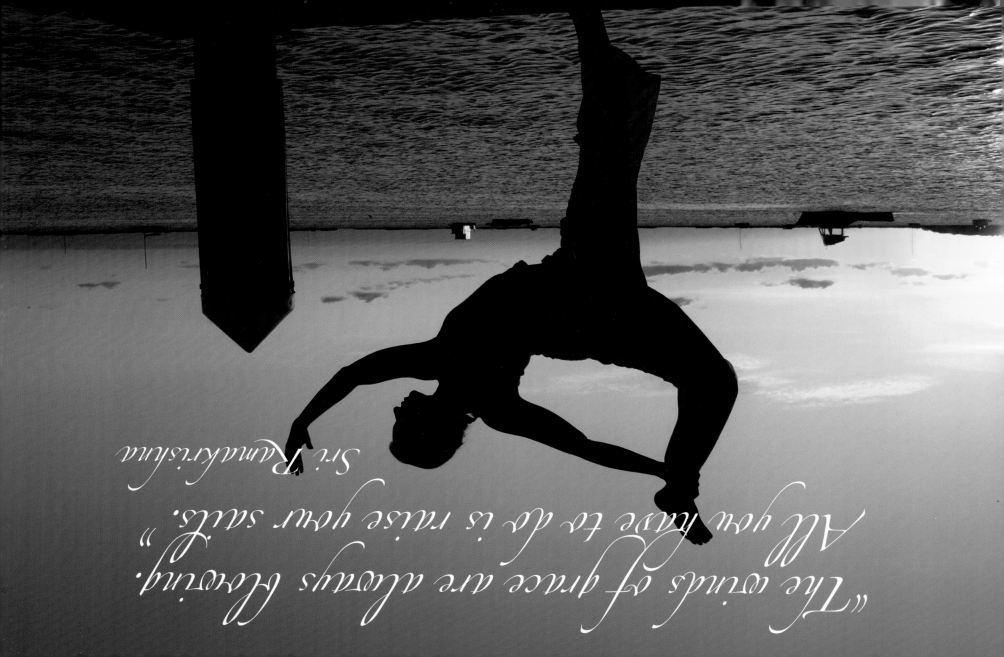

"The winds of grace are always blowing.
All you have to do is raise your sails."

Sri Ramakrishna

Restorative Postures

Legs up against the Lifelines
Reclined Spinal Twist
Corpse Pose

In this go, go, go culture that we live in, it is easy to neglect finding balance within our lives. By choosing a sailing lifestyle we embrace this need for balance; giving ourselves permission to set sail and enjoy the simplicity, the solitude and the wholeness that nature has to offer. Within our practice it is also important to balance. After doing a vigorous practice of standing postures and deep stretches, it is imperative that you include one or more of the following restorative postures. These are also great postures to do if you really don't feel like practicing at all, as they soothe the body and refresh the mind.

Legs up against the lifelines
viparita karani

This is a great pose that can be done anytime you want to relax.

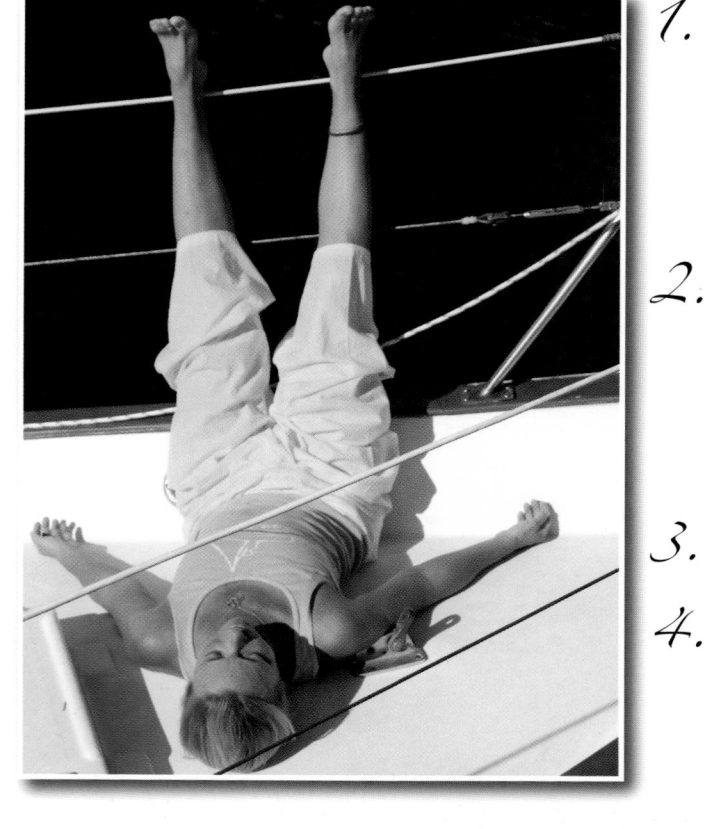

1. Begin by sitting very close to the toe rail and roll over bringing your legs up onto the lifelines.

2. The tighter your hamstrings are, the further away from the toe rail your sit bones will be.

3. Relax and breathe.

4. After a while, allow your legs to fall apart, letting gravity take over and giving your inner thighs a nice stretch.

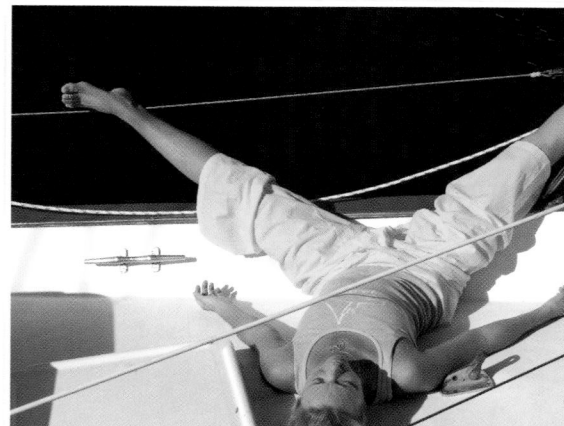

breathe

This pose can also replace any forward folds for those with extremely tight hamstrings, giving them support while stretching, and keeping the lower back aligned and protected.

Reclined Spinal Twist

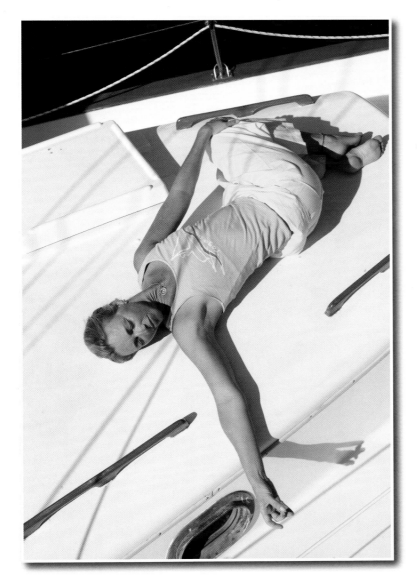

1. Begin by lying on your back.

2. Extend your arms out to the sides.

3. Bring your knees into your chest and then drop them to one side, looking to the other.

4. Switch sides.

be mindful

"Forsake all inhibitions. Pursue thy dreams!"
Walt Whitman

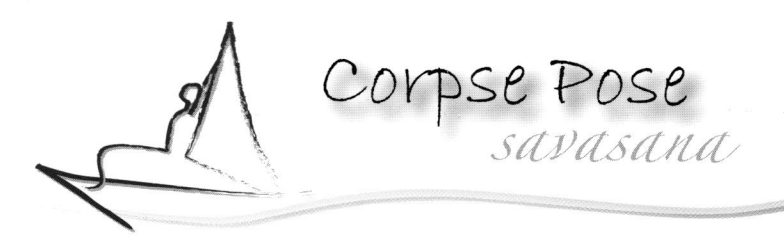

Corpse Pose
savasana

This pose is not only vital to each practice, but quite possibly the most challenging for many who find it difficult to simply rest.

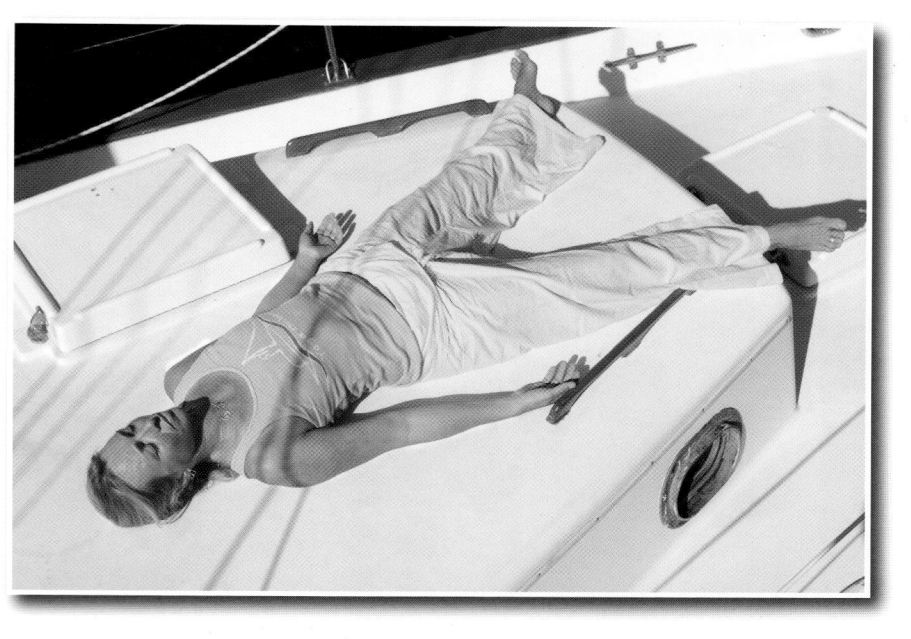

At the end of each practice, find a place that is comfortable to lie down with legs apart, arms slightly to the side with your palms up. Close your eyes and relax the body (this might be in your berth or in the shade on deck). Again, focus on the breath and completely surrender the body to gravity and the movement of the boat. Do not let the sounds of the water or of your boat distract you – rather, let them be a part of your practice.

surrender

After being in *savasana* for 5 to 10 minutes, begin to slowly bring your awareness back to your surroundings. Notice the sounds of the water against the boat, notice the rhythm of your breath, notice what you are noticing. Gently begin to move your body, beginning with your fingers and toes. Roll over onto your right side with the knees pulled in, eventually finding your way back into a comfortable cross legged position (*sukasana*), completing the circle.

AUM/OM

A (sounds like a in fall)

U (sounds like oo in moo)

M (gentle closing of the lips)

SILENCE follows

AUM is the universal sound. The beginning sound. The ending sound. It is the sound from which all other sounds emanate. It is said that all sounds in the universe are found between the A and the U. There is a certain vibration that happens when one chants this particular sanskrit word, a vibration that connects us with the Universal Oneness, a vibration that creates a sense of peace and calmness within.

To chant AUM, begin deep near the root chakra with the A. As the sound moves up through the chakra system it transforms into the U near the throat chakra and as it continues up and into the third eye, the M or ending sound begins naturally with a gentle closing of the lips. The fourth sound that is given reverence to when chanting AUM is the sound of silence.

Listen the next time you are under sail and see if you can hear the sound that is Creation.

See page 77 for information on the chakra system.

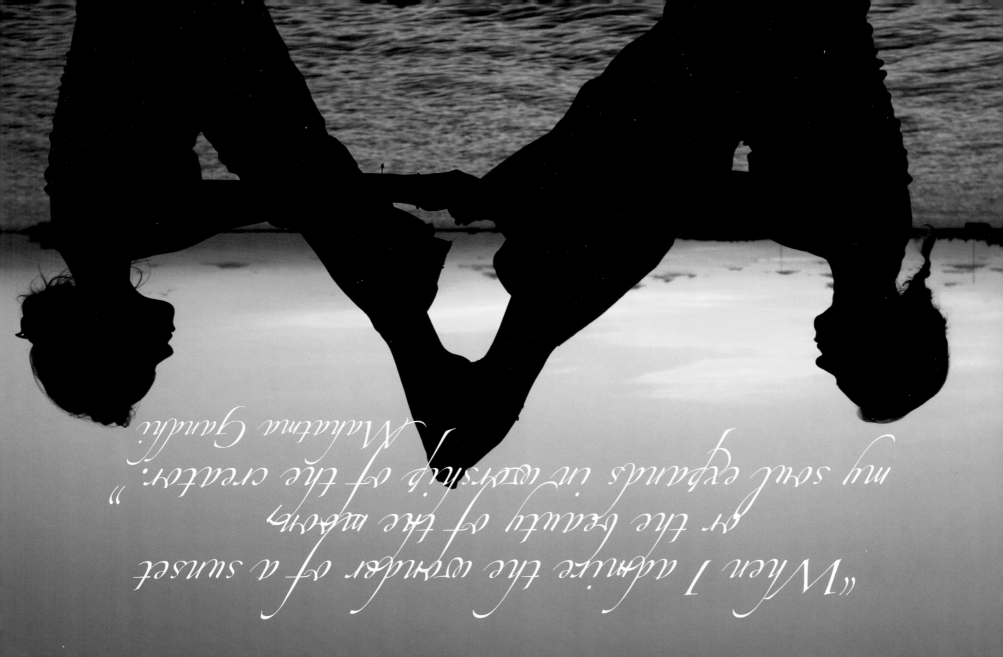

"When I admire the wonder of a sunset or the beauty of the moon, my soul expands in worship of the creator." Mahatma Gandhi

Putting it all together

Through sequencing in the order in which the book was presented your body is able to open and lengthen fully, reducing the risk of injuries. Beginning with sun salutations, moving into standing postures, backbends, seated postures and finally to your restorative postures, the muscles are able to fully warm up, lengthen and then rest. As you learn the postures, listen to your body for new and creative ways to sequence within each area.

Boat Salutations
Standing Postures
Backbends
Seated Postures
Restorative Postures

Sun salutations are traditionally done at sunrise and sunset. While practicing one afternoon traveling up the ICW in Florida on a 28' Columbia (s/v Short Story), we discovered that it worked best to split the sun salutation into two separate parts, modifying the traditional salutation for our boat salutation. In the first part, the mast was used for support; the small space at the bow was just big enough for a full plank, for the second half of the salutation.

Boat Salutations

Each movement corresponds with the breath. The inhales open and expand the body, while the exhales contract or close the body. When we do sun salutations, we allow the breath to move the body naturally. Each pose can be held for 5-10 breaths if you choose. Repeat each sequence 3-5 times. If you are practicing on the beach or a dock, combine these two sequences by stepping back into plank pose after your standing forward fold *(step 5)*.

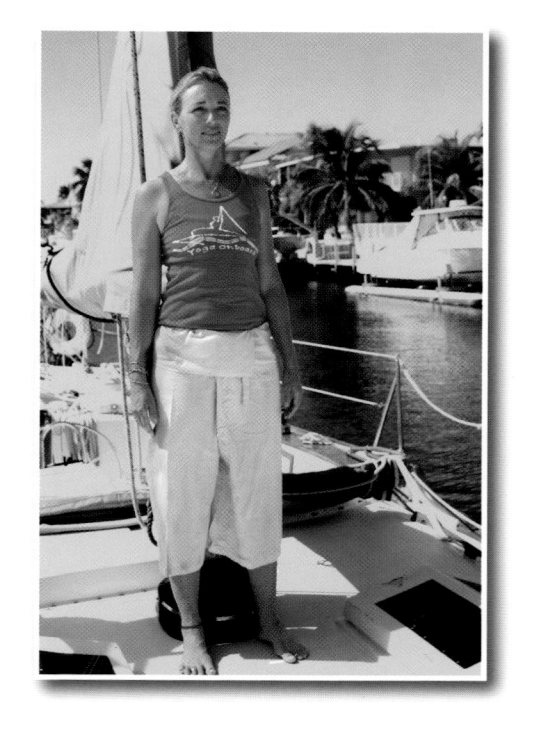 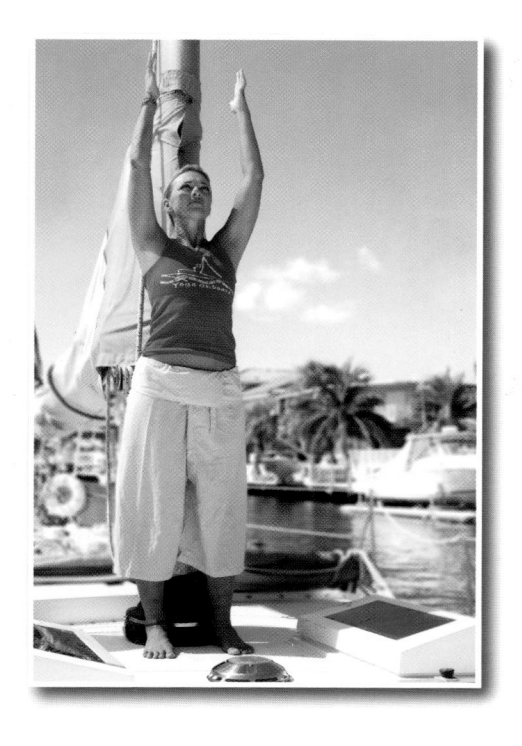 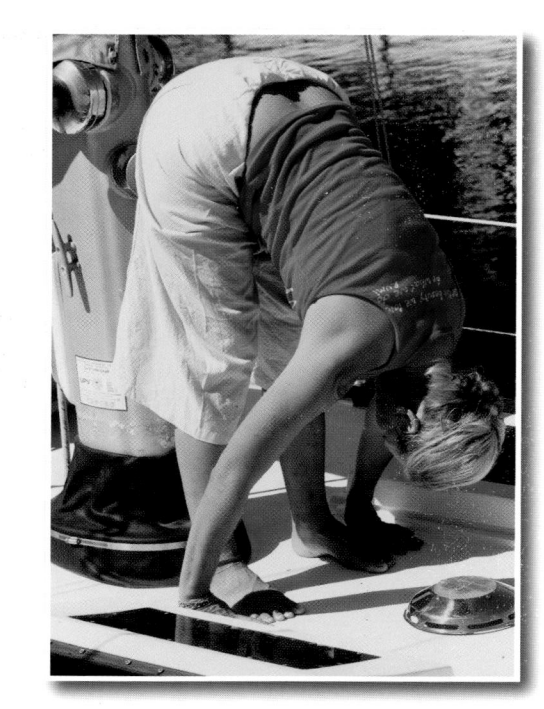

1. Begin in mountain pose.

2. Inhale into extended mountain pose.

3. Exhale into standing forward fold.

4. Inhale half way up to lengthen the spine.

5. Exhale as you return to standing forward fold.

6. Inhale, reach the arms out and up into extended mountain pose.

7. Exhale into mountain pose.

1. Begin in plank pose, inhale.
2. As you exhale, slowly lower into four limb staff pose.
3. Inhale into upward facing dog or cobra.

4. Exhale into downward facing dog.
5. To repeat, inhale into plank pose.

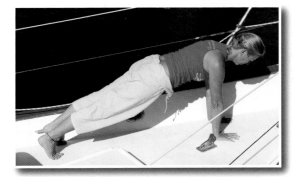

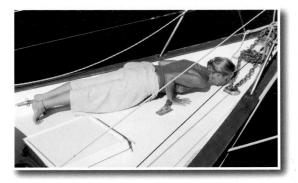

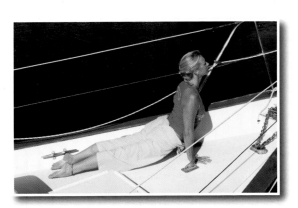

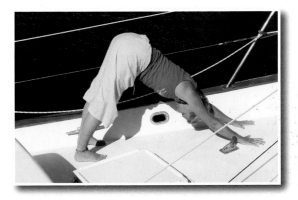

Modifications:

For those that have not built their core strength or are dealing with any physical conditions, drop the knees down for plank pose, keeping the back straight. As you exhale, drop your chest and chin between your hands, then drop your belly and hips. By doing this you will protect your lower back while increasing the strength in your core and upper body.

Standing Postures

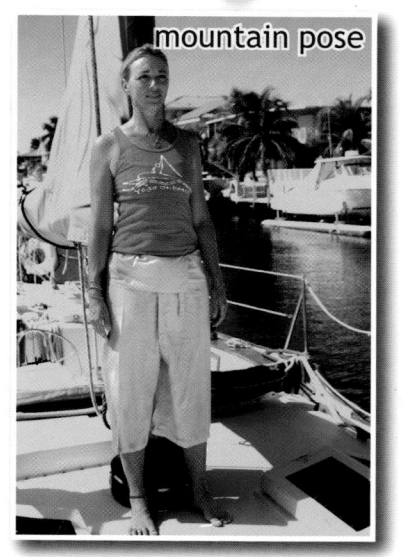
mountain pose

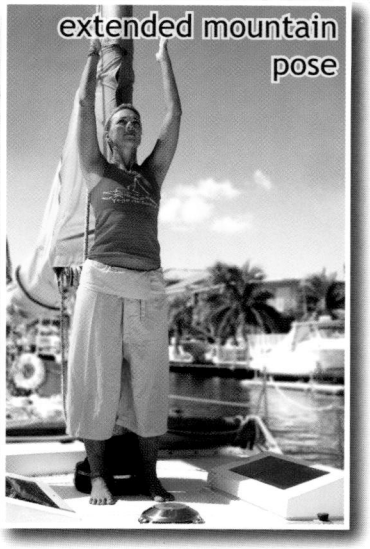
extended mountain pose

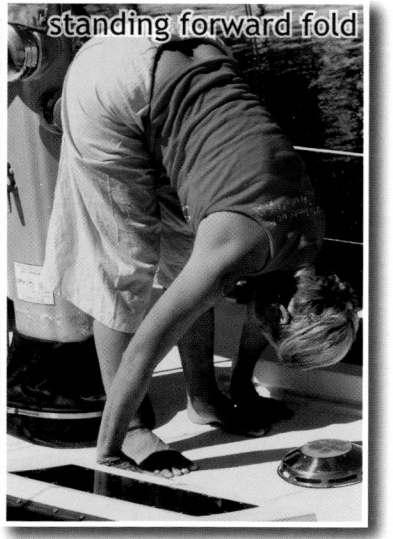
standing forward fold

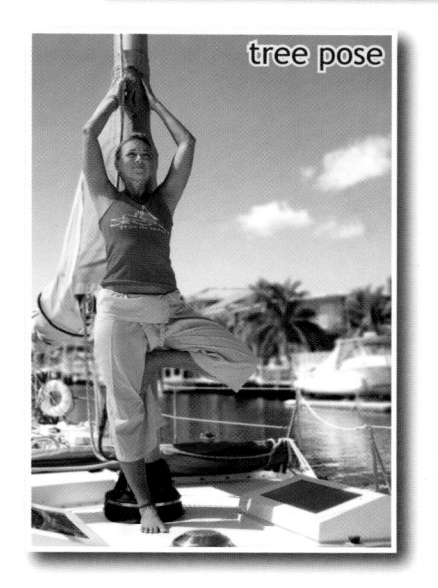
tree pose

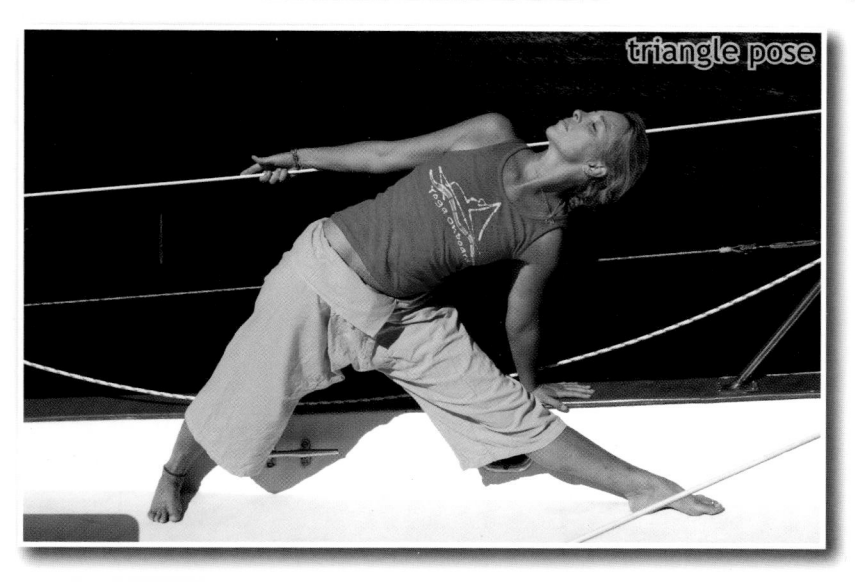
triangle pose

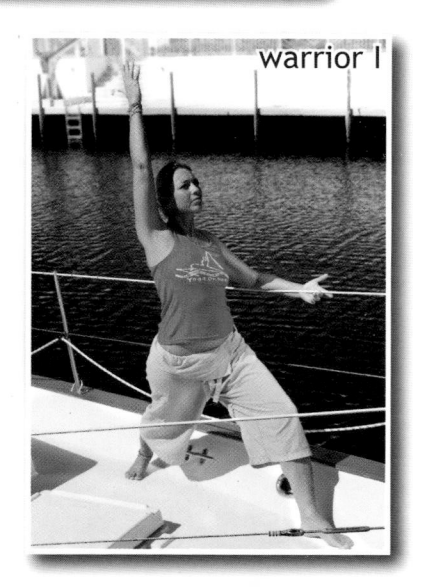
warrior I

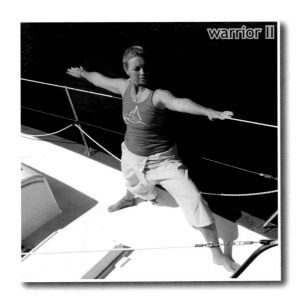
warrior II

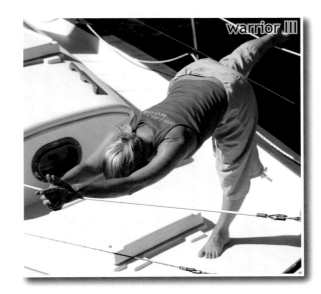
warrior III

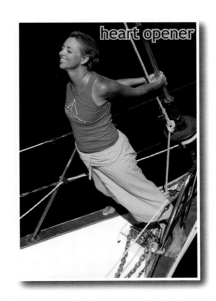
heart opener

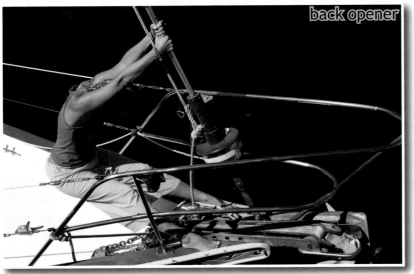
back opener

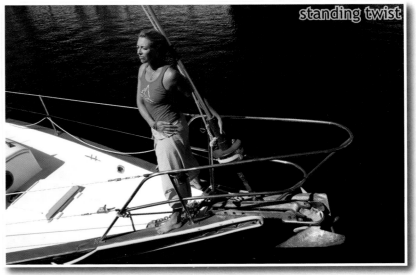
standing twist

67

Backbends

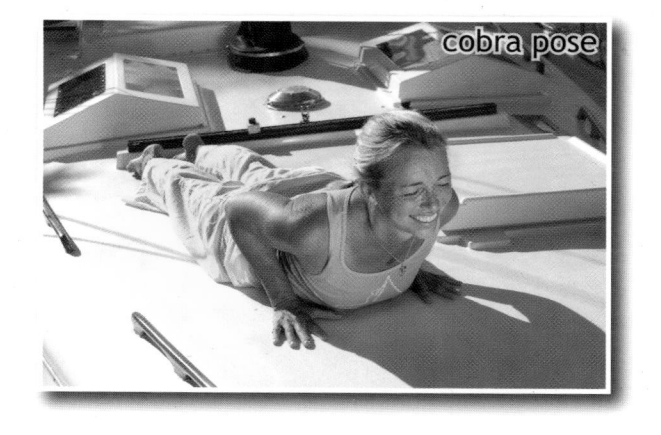

cobra pose

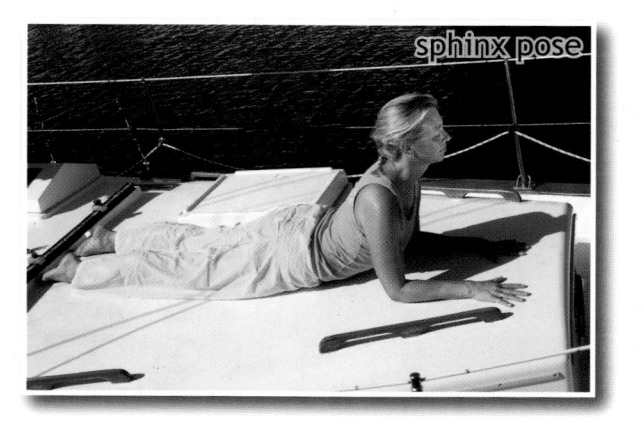

sphinx pose

after backbends

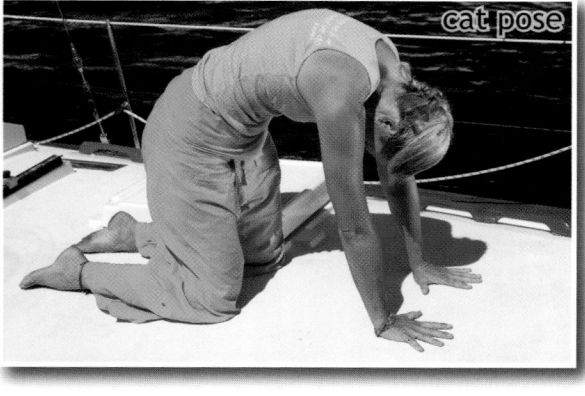

cow pose

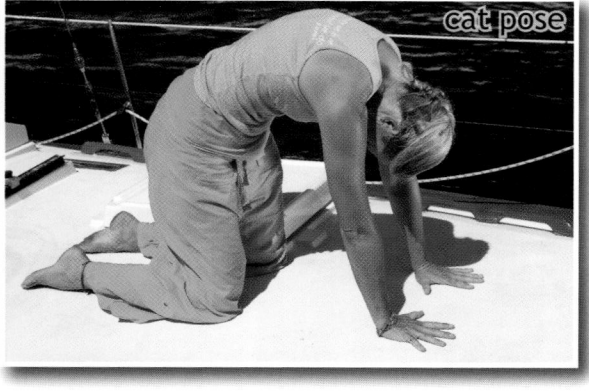

cat pose

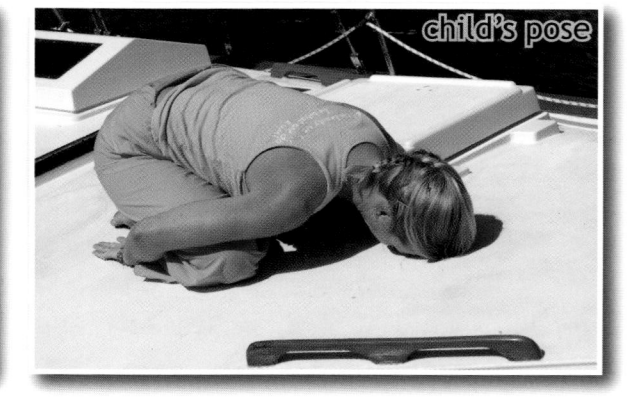

child's pose

Seated Postures

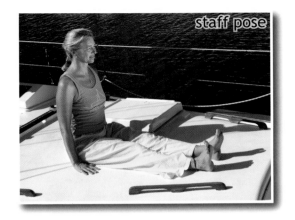
staff pose

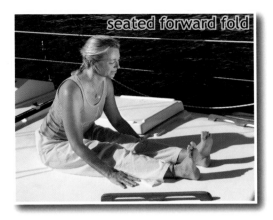
seated forward fold

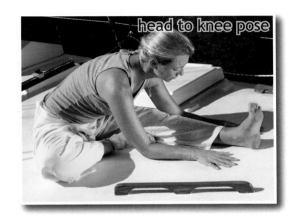
head to knee pose

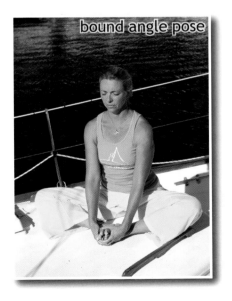
bound angle pose

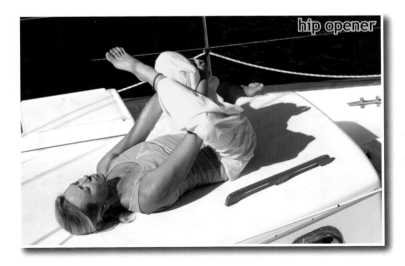
hip opener

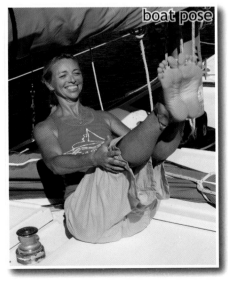
boat pose

Restorative Postures

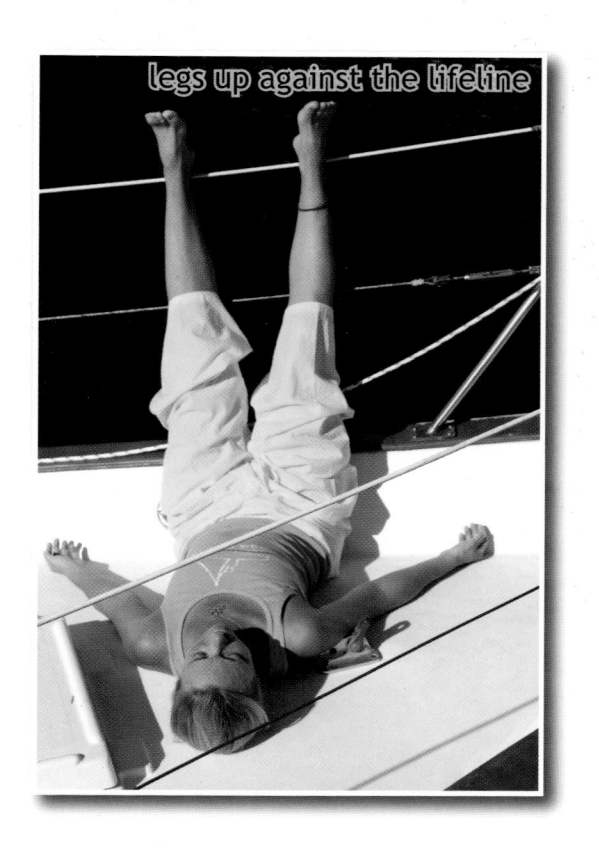

legs up against the lifeline

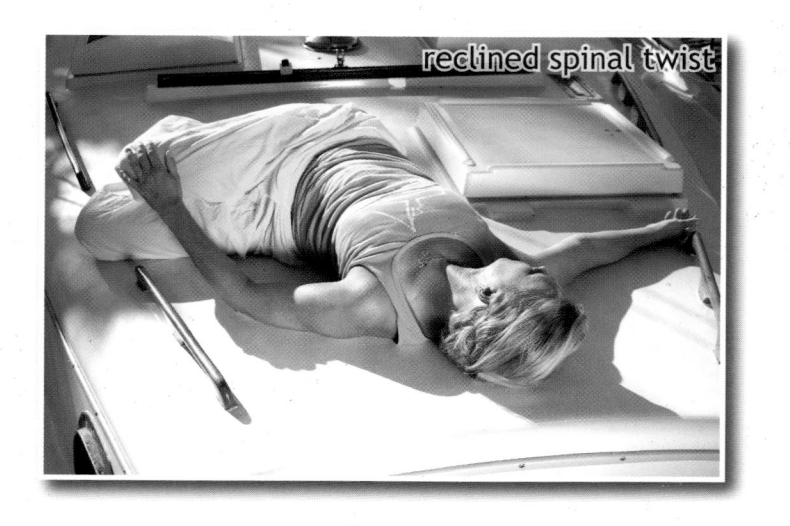

reclined spinal twist

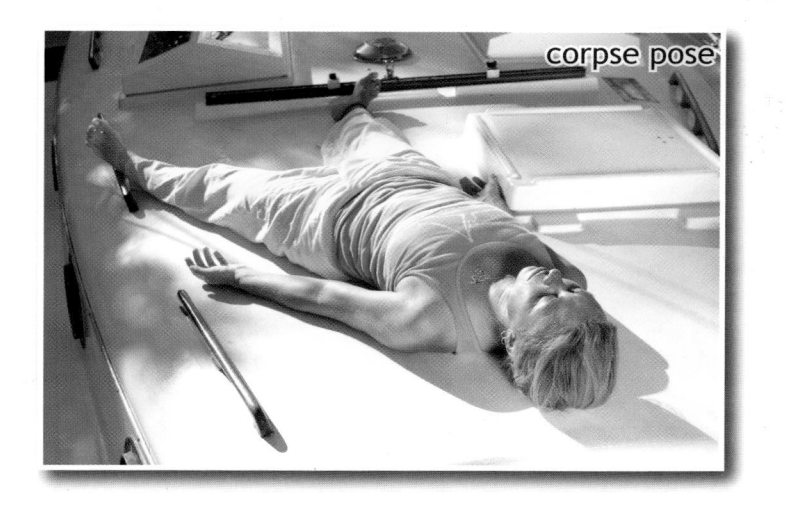

corpse pose

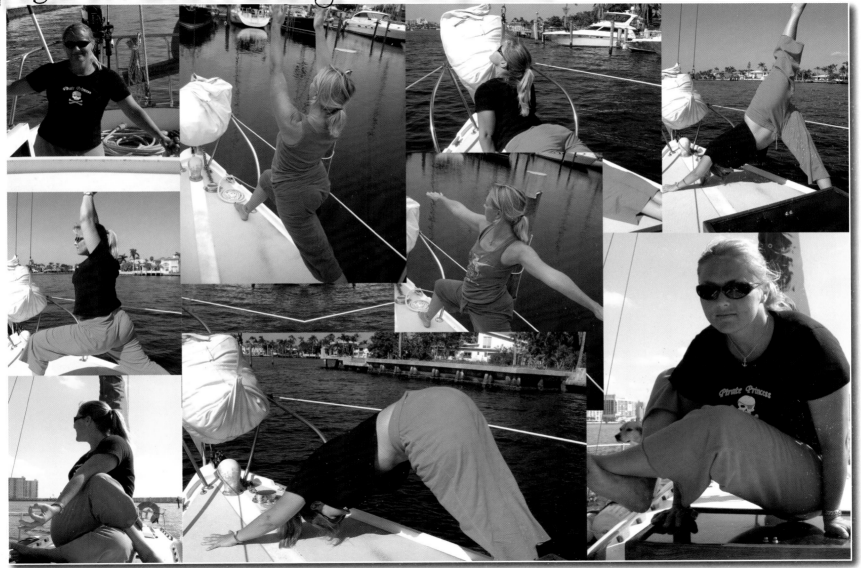

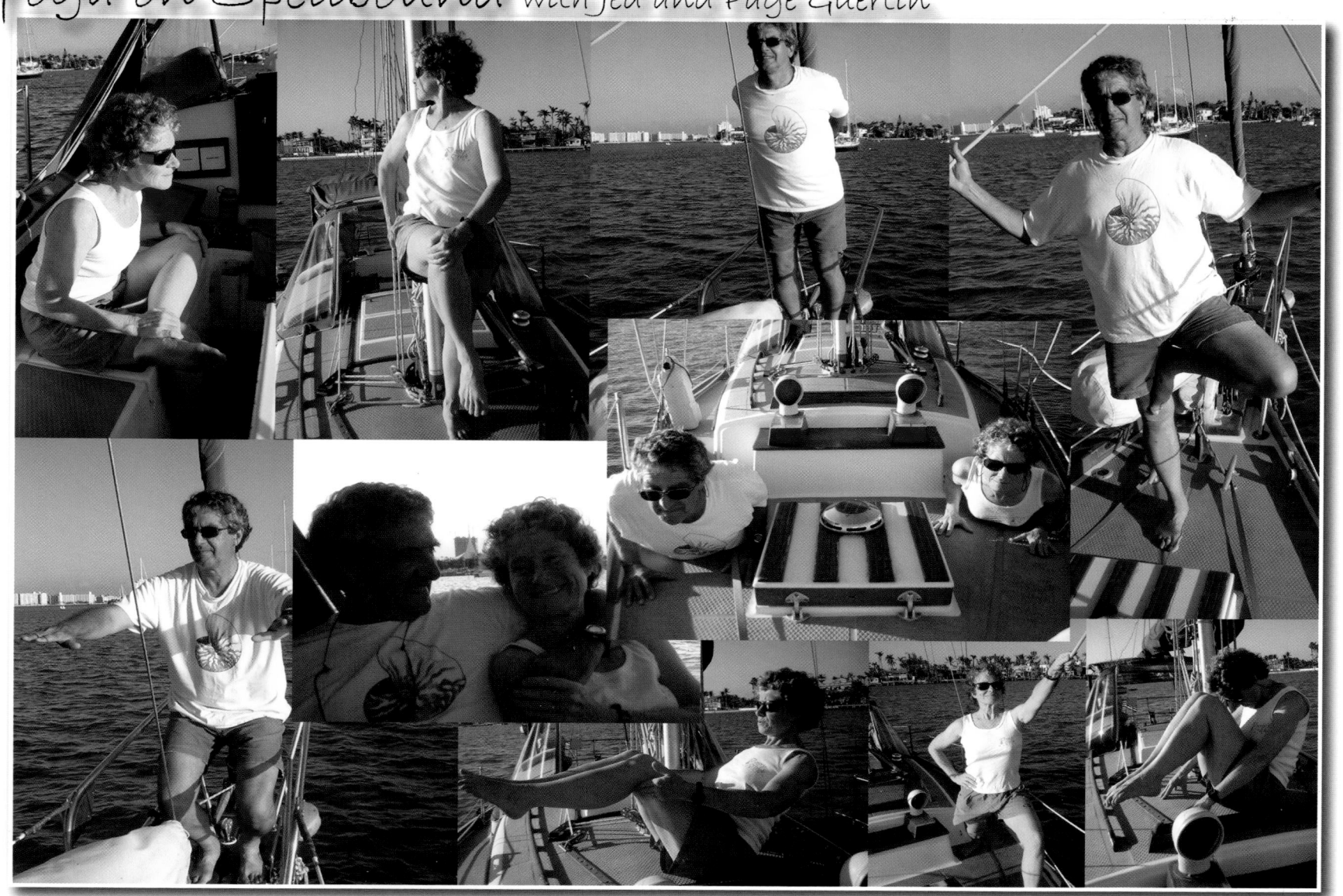

Yoga on Spellbound with Jed and Page Guertin

Yoga on Dutch Love with Kim

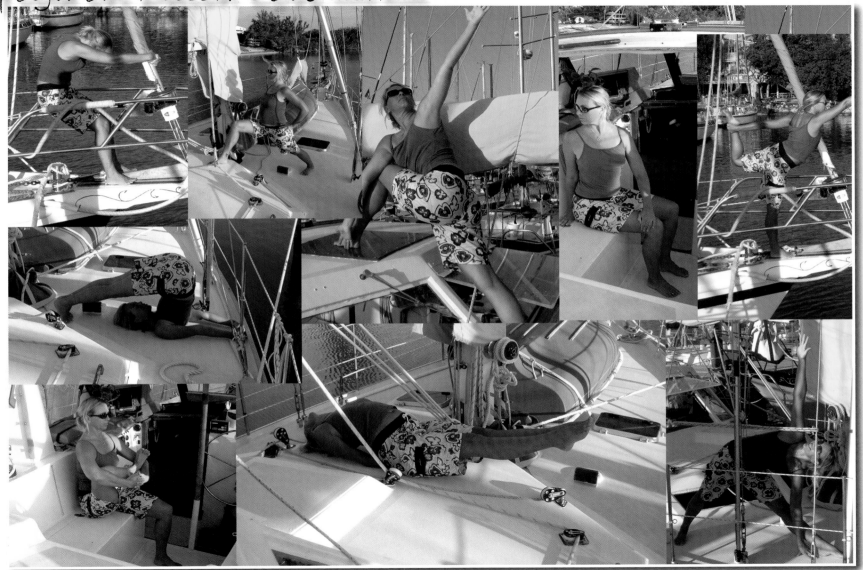

Ending Thoughts

We have tapped into the surface of yoga asana which is only 1/8 of what yoga is all about. I encourage you to explore more deeply this ancient practice. There are many great books, DVDs and teachers out there. Next time you are in port, find a yoga class to attend. Working with an instructor is invaluable in building your practice.

The information shared here can also be taken to the beach or the docks. Grab your mat, a large towel or Mexican blanket and enjoy the different sensations that practicing in various places has to offer. Just notice how each place creates a completely new practice for you. Notice any emotions that arise, how your ability to focus may shift and how different each pose feels. My philosophy is that how we "be" on the mat is how we "be" in life. What I mean by this is the way we approach our practice is a direct reflection of how we take on life. Are you distracted easily by what is going on around you? How committed are you? Are you willing to slow down and notice the little details, or do you rush through things, just to get them done? Are you willing to show compassion for yourself as well as for others? Every lesson learned while practicing can be applied to some area of your life.

Yoga is truly a gift of life, of the realization of the beauty surrounding us. As sailors we live within the most magnificent part of this beauty – in and of the sea. With a devoted yoga practice not only will your appreciation for this grow, but a sense of awareness to the breath and the physical body will deepen, encouraging a healthier and more vibrant life.

I would like to express my deepest gratitude to my friends, old and new, my family – I love you - and to the entire Yoga Onboard team without whom this project would have remained just an idea. I believe that each experience we have and each relationship we choose, creates the person who we are.

Growing up in a small community has given me the opportunity to realize the importance of forming lifetime bonds. To all of you who have found a place in my heart and will forever be considered "family" in Idaho, Florida and Mexico – thank you. The quiet inspiration you have given me is invaluable. And to those of you with whom my path has not yet crossed, I look forward to sharing time with you.

I bow humbly to my guides and teachers throughout the years. Mary Jostes who introduced me to the path I am now on, the Dead Monkeys who held my hand, wiped my tears and rolled with laughter as we all grew in leaps and bounds through our years together, Wilbert Alix who introduced me to the way of the shaman and Gaia Buddha, founder of Synergy Center for Yoga and the Healing Arts, my home studio. However, my two greatest teachers are my children Erika and Dallas.

There are no words that express the expanse of gratitude that lies in my heart for my parents and my brother, who without their realization, have inspired me to strive to be the person I am today.

And finally to the Yoga Onboard team - Gino, for the inspiration to act NOW. Captain Harman, for his encouragement and support. Rigo, who started out as my student and grew into my teacher. Melanie, who inspires me daily. Liz, for her key lime pies! Julia, for always being there. Melissa, for her kind and gentle support. And Suzanne, who, through her words, never ending support and unconditional love, opened my heart, lifted me up and led me to Grace.

I would also like to thank Calypso Sailing of Key Largo for the use of their vessel for our photo shoot. Raychel Brown and Jody Lipkin for believing in me, and Jed and Page for their enthusiasm and support.

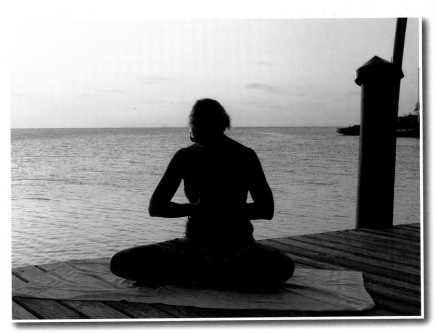

The divine sweetness that dwells deep within me, acknowledges and honors the eternal light that shines from deep within you.

We are One.

Namaste.

Namaste

This word can be taken to mean any of the following:

- The Spirit in me meets the same Spirit in you.
- I greet that place where you and I are one.
- I salute the Divine in you.
- I salute the Light of God in you.
- I bow to the Divine in you.
- I recognize that within each of us is a place where Divinity dwells, and when we are in that place, we are One.

By saying the word namaste, we recognize the equality of all, and pay honor to the sacredness and interconnection of all, as well as to the source of that interconnection.

Namaste is generally said at the end of a yoga class. It is also used as a greeting. The palms of the hands are brought together in front of the heart center or forehead with a simple bow. This action can also be used to symbolize the actual word.

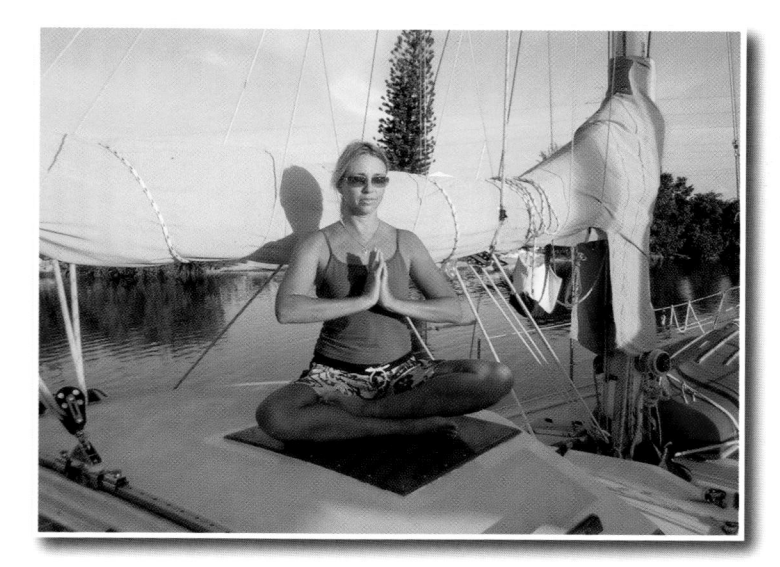

Our Energy System - The Chakras

The Chakras are a system of energy 'wheels' that are located along our energetic spine, beginning near the perineum and moving upward to the top of the head. Each chakra is associated with a color and physical as well as emotional energies.

When practicing the physical postures we want to keep the spine - the physical as well as the 'energetic' spine as long and straight as possible, enabling the energy to flow freely. This assists us in achieving that place of ease and comfort within each pose.

THE SEVEN CHAKRAS:

NAME	LOCATION	PHYSICAL ASSOCIATIONS	EMOTIONAL ASSOCIATIONS
1st or Root	perineum/pelvic floor	lower extremities, immune system	survival, belief systems
2nd or Spleen	just below the belly button	sexual organs, bladder, hip area	money, sex and creativity
3rd or Solar Plexis	2-3 inches above the belly button	abdomen, kidney, liver, adrenal glands, spleen	personal power, trust, intuitive powers
4th or Heart	heart center	heart, circulatory system, lungs, shoulders, arms	love, anger, loneliness, forgiveness, compassion
5th or Throat	throat	throat, thyroid, neck, mouth	personal expression, following one's dream, judgement
6th or Third Eye	between the brows	brain, nervous system, eyes, ears, nose, pineal and pituitary glands	truth, emotional intelligence
7th or Crown	top of the head	muscular and skeletal systems, skin	values, ethics, and courage, faith, wisdom

Karma Yoga and Shake-A-Leg Miami

Revisiting the branches of yoga (p.11), one branch in particular is very important in my life. Through karma yoga I have learned what it means to be a part of the never ending cycle of giving and receiving with no motive other than to uplift the lives of others. One way to give in this manner is to volunteer or perform community service. I would like to take this opportunity to introduce you to an organization that I am currently involved with.

Shake-A-Leg Miami is a non-profit organization originally created to offer sailing to disabled persons. This amazing organization has grown into a phenomenal institution where disabled persons of all ages as well as disadvantaged children and families come together for water sports activities, academic, art and computer programs. Also offered are many community activities including but not limited to sailing classes and regattas. The structure is supported by volunteers of all physical abilities. Shake-A-Leg, its staff and students have brought me much joy.

If you are ever in the Miami area please drop by for a visit, offer to volunteer or participate in one of the many social activities offered. I also encourage you to find a way to practice karma yoga wherever you happen to be. I know that cruisers are known for pitching in to assist local communities which are in need. This is one of the many reasons why I am proud to be a part of the sailing community.

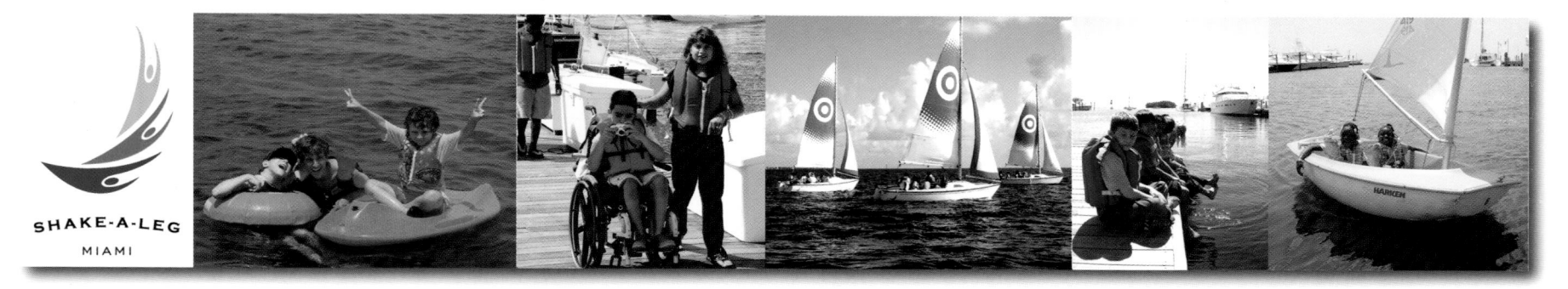

"The beauty and charm of selfless love and service should not die away from the face of the earth. The world should know that a life of dedication is possible, that a life inspired by love and service to humanity is possible. Through selfless action we can eradicate the ego that conceals the Self. Detached, selfless action leads to liberation. Such action is not just work, it is karma yoga."   *The Hindu Saint Mata Amritanandamayi*

Index

Index

Main Reference Materials:

Iyengar, B.K.S..
Light on Yoga

Swenson, David
Ashtanga Yoga "The Practice Manual"

Sri Swami Satchidananda,
Translation and Commentary by
The Yoga Sutras of Patanjali

Myss, Caroline
Anatomy of The Spirit